T0327074

Handbook of Equine Parasite Control

Handbook of Equine Parasite Control

Second Edition

Martin K. Nielsen, DVM, PhD, Dipl. ACVM
Associate Professor and Schlaikjer Professor
Department of Veterinary Science
M.H. Gluck Equine Research Center
University of Kentucky
Lexington, Kentucky, USA

Craig R. Reinemeyer, DVM, PhD, Dipl. ACVM
President, East Tennessee Clinical Research
Rockwood, Tennessee, USA

WILEY Blackwell

Registered Office
John Wiley & Sons, Inc., 111 River Street, Hoboken, NJ 07030, USA

Editorial Office
111 River Street, Hoboken, NJ 07030, USA

For details of our global editorial offices, customer services, and more information about Wiley products visit us at www.wiley.com.

Wiley also publishes its books in a variety of electronic formats and by print-on-demand. Some content that appears in standard print versions of this book may not be available in other formats.

Library of Congress Cataloging-in-Publication Data

Names: Nielsen, Martin Krarup, 1972–, author | Reinemeyer, Craig Robert, 1952–, author
Title: Handbook of equine parasite control / Martin K. Nielsen, Craig R. Reinemeyer.
Description: Second edition. | Hoboken, NJ : John Wiley & Sons, Inc., 2018. | Craig R. Reinemeyer's
   name appears first in the previous edition. | Includes bibliographical references and index. |
Identifiers: LCCN 2018000457 (print) | LCCN 2018001338 (ebook) | ISBN 9781119382805 (pdf) |
   ISBN 9781119382812 (epub) | ISBN 9781119382782 (cloth)
Subjects: | MESH: Horse Diseases–therapy | Parasitic Diseases, Animal–prevention & control
Classification: LCC SF959.P37 (ebook) | LCC SF959.P37 (print) | NLM SF 959.P37 | DDC 636.1–dc23
LC record available at https://lccn.loc.gov/2018000457

Cover design: Martin K Nielsen
Cover images: Top: *Parascaris* spp. eggs obtained from a single female worm (Photo courtesy: Maci Stephens). Middle: Icelandic colts on pasture (Photo courtesy: Shaila Sigsgaard).
Bottom: *Anoplocephala perfoliata* eggs recovered from a gravid proglottid (Photo courtesy: Jamie Norris).

Set in 10/12pt Warnock by SPi Global, Pondicherry, India

10 9 8 7 6 5 4 3 2 1

Dedication

We dedicate this second edition to Dr. Eugene T. Lyons and his career-long assistant Ms. Sharon C. Tolliver, who both passed away shortly before this second edition went into print. They were passionate equine parasitologists, good friends, and highly respected by colleagues around the world. They both worked at the University of Kentucky for over 50 years and their contributions to equine parasitology are unmatched. They are by far the most cited authors in this book. Dr. Lyons described the life cycles of Strongyloides westeri, Thelazia lacrymalis, *and* Strongylus vulgaris. *He virtually tested and evaluated every single anthelmintic product that ever made it to the equine market, and he diligently documented the progression of anthelmintic resistance in equine parasites. He published over 300 research articles. Sharon was his right and left hands through all of this. She was one of the world's few experts on identifying equine helminth specimens, and she herself contributed to over 200 seminal publications in equine parasitology. It was a privilege to know and work with the two of them. They were both equine parasitologists* par excellence *and their passing really marks the end of an era. The discipline of veterinary parasitology is diminished by their absence, but their spirits and contributions linger on – as evidenced by this book.*

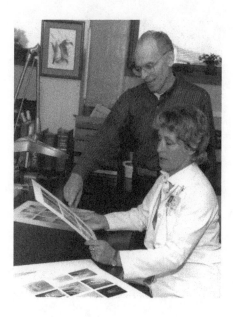

Contents

List of Contributors

Dave Leathwick PhD
AgResearch Grasslands
Palmerston North
New Zealand

Christian Sauermann PhD
AgResearch Grasslands
Palmerston North
New Zealand

Preface to the First Edition

This book was conceived through the authors' realization that equine practitioners were not likely to achieve competence in evidence-based parasite control (EBPC) by reading journal-length articles or by attending a few hours of continuing education. Like any clinical skill set, parasite control must be grounded solidly in theory, practiced with thoughtful application, and continuously assessed and improved. Most new clinical skills, such as surgical procedures or diagnostic algorithms, represent variations of basic proficiencies or knowledge already held by practitioners, who can also turn to local mentors for advice and support. In contrast, the private sector harbors few, if any, experts in equine parasitology who can impart mastery of the principles of EBPC.

Evidence-based parasite control is a relatively new development in equine medicine, but similar principles have been applied for decades by small ruminant practitioners in Europe and the southern hemisphere. In these locales, parasitic challenges to indigenous livestock are prevalent and extreme. Near-total anthelmintic resistance by certain parasites (*e.g.*, *Haemonchus contortus*) has rendered practical control of these highly pathogenic nematodes nearly impossible, with severe economic consequences for the sheep and goat industries on multiple continents. In comparison, equine cyathostomins (small strongyles) have demonstrated resistance to one or more anthelmintic classes for nearly four decades, but these nematodes are modest pathogens under most circumstances. The authors and other veterinary parasitologists have been disseminating EBPC recommendations for many years, but equine practitioners have been relatively unreceptive to these messages until very recently. The impetus for this changed attitude is uncertain, but it seems to be associated with the contemporary detection of anthelmintic resistance in some populations of *Parascaris equorum*. Mere demonstration of resistance in a second group of equine parasites is not likely the major threat perceived by practitioners. Rather, it could be the hard evidence that macrocyclic lactone anthelmintics, previously considered bullet-proof panaceas in horses, are also vulnerable to nematode resistance.

Regardless of the motivation, equine practitioners now seem uniquely receptive to EBPC, and this book represents our attempt to address that interest and to fill the need with practical advice and logical recommendations. Most veterinary textbooks organize and discuss related facts, and then present recommendations for the logical application of that knowledge in clinical situations. This handbook has an additional objective that is far more daunting. The authors face the challenge of changing a mindset; of overcoming four decades of tradition, literally tens of millions of episodes of implementation, and competing recommendations from the marketing departments of every pharmaceutical company with a horse in the race. Change is painful but necessary, and progress in parasite control will be measured one practitioner and one horse owner at a time. As Darwin famously observed, "It is not the strongest of the species that survives, nor the most intelligent that survives. It is the one that is the most adaptable to change." The worms have been changing since the dawn of effective anthelmintic therapy; now it's our turn.

We have not included an exhaustive collection of references in this book, because busy practitioners have neither the time nor the means to delve deeper into relevant literature. In addition, we readily acknowledge the irony that many of our "evidence-based" recommendations have minimal scientific support at present.

So until more definitive proof is published, some practices clearly represent "stop digging" advice. (This term is derived from the adage that when you find yourself in a hole, the first thing to do is stop digging.) It is often a greater management challenge to convince people to stop doing the wrong thing than it is for them to adopt correct measures.

Our primary goal is to teach, and we believe that training in EBPC is best done by vet-side mentors. Accordingly, we beg the reader's indulgence whenever our tone becomes informal or even casual. This merely reflects our teaching styles.

October, 2012

Martin K. Nielsen
Craig R. Reinemeyer

Preface to the Second Edition

"Parasite control is confusing." "There are so many opinions out there." "What's wrong with continuing to follow our historical practices?" Statements like these are commonly made by people who reach out to us with questions about this topic. While we understand these frustrations, they are really unnecessary and they are the main reasons for writing this book, which now emerges in its Second Edition. Equine parasitology is a very small research field with a limited number of scientists involved across the world. One would not expect a lot of new information to be developed in just a handful of years. Nonetheless, a substantial amount of new knowledge has been generated and relevant technology has emerged since the First Edition of this book was published in 2013. Thus, we found it timely to update the contents and publish a Second Edition.

It has been our ambition from the very beginning to make this a practical book, written in straightforward language, and we have attempted to retain this style in the Second Edition. The case scenarios near the end of the book serve as a testament to this ambition. Having said that, we realize that the text may appear somewhat academic to some, and we make extensive use of scientific-style references throughout. Although the majority of readers are unlikely to look up references and read scientific papers, we know from experience with the First Edition that a proportion will do this. Therefore, we have expanded the reference lists with papers published within the last five years. Veterinarians who are members of American Association of Equine Practitioners (AAEP) or British Equine Veterinary Association (BEVA) will notice that the authors have published several review papers in the journal *Equine Veterinary Education*, which is distributed to the membership of both associations. Thus, there is direct access to more in-depth information there. We consider the citation of published references as a healthy and objective exercise, which helps us to avoid making unsupported and sometimes misleading assumptions. In a world where any kind of information can be disseminated globally in a matter of seconds, we believe that basing recommendations on credible and peer-reviewed evidence is the only responsible approach for a publication such as this. Veterinary textbooks and the scientific literature are full of examples of statements that are repeated through generations. In the end, no one remembers where the statement originated or why a specific practice was initiated. When the literature is searched meticulously, it is often found that a statement has been misconstrued or that it was never based on objective data to begin with. Along those lines, revisiting the literature helped us to identify some misleading and even erroneous content that appeared in the First Edition. Yes, we are also guilty of making unsubstantiated assumptions.

While we have not experienced the launch of a new anthelmintic class for equines since the First Edition was published, we have enjoyed remarkable advances on the diagnostic frontier. As a result, the diagnostic chapter (Chapter 9) has grown more than any other portion of this book. A parasitologist cannot imagine a world without our beloved fecal egg counts, and despite their old school nature, we can conclude that they are here to stay. In fact, they remain the foundation of good evidence-based parasite control. The diagnostic chapter contains an expanded discussion of interpretation of fecal egg counts, with special emphasis on accuracy and precision. Furthermore, this edition has devoted an entire chapter to anthelmintic resistance. We continue to see more and more resistance across the world, and this chapter features two sets of heat maps summarizing all reported findings of anthelmintic resistance in cyathostomin and *Parascaris* spp. parasites.

Some exciting developments have evolved since 2013. One of these is the use of computer modeling to predict the dynamics of equine parasite infections and anthelmintic resistance development. These tools allow us to investigate the principles of these complicated biological phenomena without the need to involve live animals in tedious, expensive, and frequently inconclusive research. This book also includes contributions from two leading scientists in the field of computer modeling: Dr. Dave Leathwick and Dr. Christian Sauermann from AgResearch, New Zealand. They have generously provided model simulation outputs which illustrate important biological principles in equine parasitology.

Other unique features in this Second Edition include the addition of new clinical case scenarios near the end of the book. These are all based on actual cases that we have encountered through the years. The book also features a glossary of technical and scientific terms that appear in the book. Hopefully, this glossary will increase the understanding of readers who are not veterinarians or parasitologists. Finally, a large number of new images have been added.

We realize that we just represent another opinion about parasitology; we might even be adding to the confusion about these topics. Nonetheless, our ambition is the exact opposite, and our opinions at least are based on the best possible evidence available at this time. Undoubtedly, we will need to revise some of the content again in a few years. Until then, enjoy.

June, 2018

Martin K. Nielsen
Craig R. Reinemeyer

Acknowledgements

We are deeply grateful to fellow scientists, veterinarians, horse owners, and farm managers from all over the world for asking us challenging questions about equine parasite control. They serve as an invaluable source of inspiration for this book. Sincere thanks to our friends, colleagues, and collaborators in New Zealand, Drs Dave Leathwick and Christian Sauermann, for their insightful contributions to several chapters. We warmly acknowledge Dr. Tetiana Kuzmina, Dr. Stine Jacobsen, Dr. Paul Slusarewicz, Dr. Alan Loynachan, Ms. Shaila Sigsgaard, Ms. Holli Gravatte, Mr. Jamie Norris, Ms. Maci Stephens, Ms. Faith Miller, Ms. Jennifer Bellaw, Ms. Maria Rhod, and Ms. Tina Roust for providing high quality photographs. Last, but not least, we are deeply indebted to Mr. Jamie Norris, a scientific illustrator in the making, for preparing beautiful life cycle figures and for his tireless help with digitally optimizing image quality.

Section I

Internal Parasites and Factors Affecting Their Transmission

1

Biology and Life Cycles of Equine Parasites

Life cycles are the road maps that guide parasites to their ultimate goal – propagating a subsequent generation. Some parasites follow a single, direct path to grandma's house, while yet others may travel by convoluted routes, sojourn for protracted periods at some wayside convenience, or even pick up a passenger or two. These differences represent alternate strategies for coping with the vagaries of the environment and of their eventual hosts.

A thorough knowledge of life cycles is not emphasized merely to torment veterinary students. Rather, life cycle details reveal opportunities to control parasites through chemical or management interventions, to exploit unfavorable environmental conditions, or to promote natural enemies that might act as agents of biological control. Taking advantage of these potential control opportunities will be emphasized in individual chapters in this volume.

At the root of all life cycles is a fundamental principle that distinguishes helminth parasites from other infectious agents such as viruses, bacteria, fungi, and protozoa. Through various types of clonal expansion, the latter can all amplify their numbers within a host animal. Literally millions of individual organisms may arise from infective burdens that are orders of magnitude smaller. The reproductive products of nearly all helminths, however, are required to leave the host and undergo essential change in a different location. Defecation is the most common means by which reproductive products exit the host, but a notable exception includes immature parasitic stages that are ingested by blood-sucking arthropods (*e.g.*, *Onchocerca*, *Setaria*). Most parasitic products can become infective in the environment, whereas others require intermediate hosts or vectors. Regardless, all of these essential transformations occur "outside the definitive host". Indeed, dramatic biological change is mandatory before a parasitic organism is capable of infecting a new host animal or of reinfecting the original host.

Compared to those organisms that amplify their numbers through clonal expansion, helminth disease is a numbers game. Simply put, as the number of invading parasites increases, greater tissue damage or nutrient loss results, and the range and severity of clinical signs become more extensive.

In this chapter, we propose to describe the basic life cycles of the major helminth parasites of equids. Specific control opportunities may be mentioned in this overview, but these will be discussed more fully elsewhere in the volume.

Nematodes

Superfamily Strongyloidea

The members of the Strongyloidea ("strongyles") are moderately sized, stout worms with substantial buccal capsules.

Handbook of Equine Parasite Control, Second Edition. Martin K. Nielsen and Craig R. Reinemeyer.
© 2018 John Wiley & Sons, Inc. Published 2018 by John Wiley & Sons, Inc.

The males have a copulatory bursa at the posterior end and females of all species produce eggs that are similar in appearance. Eggs of small strongyles cannot be differentiated microscopically from those of large strongyles, and the only practical method of differentiation (other than molecular approaches) is through coproculture. The strongyloids of horses all have direct life cycles; intermediate or paratenic hosts are never used (Figure 1.1).

Strongyloid eggs pass in feces and hatch in favorable environmental conditions of moisture, temperature, and

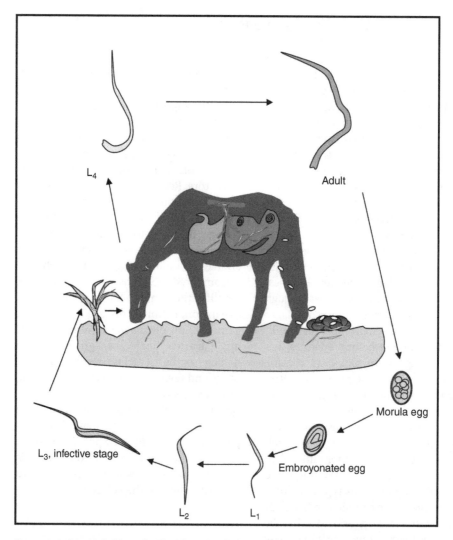

Figure 1.1 Strongyle life cycle. The life cycle of strongyle parasites. Parasitic stages can be seen above the horse and preparasitic stages below it. Fertilized eggs are shed by adult females in the cecum and colon, and excreted to the environment in the feces. Here, the eggs hatch and a first-stage larva (L_1) emerges. The L_1 then molts to L_2 in the feces. Another molt gives rise to the L_3, which retains its L_2 cuticle and thus has a double-layered sheath. The L_3 leaves the fecal pat and migrates on to forage, where it is ingested by a horse. Inside the horse, the L_3 exsheathes and invades the mucosa of the large intestine. Large strongyles (*Strongylus* spp.) undergo extensive migration in various organs of the horse, while cyathostomins encyst in the mucosal lining of the large intestine. After returning to the large intestinal lumen, the worms reach sexual maturity and start shedding eggs.

oxygenation. All species exhibit three sequential larval stages, first (L_1), second (L_2), and third (L_3). The L_1 and L_2 stages feed on organic material in the environment, but the third stage develops within the sheath of the L_2. This protective covering helps L_3s to resistant environmental conditions, but it has no oral opening, so third stage larvae are unable to ingest nutrients. The L_3 is the infective stage for all strongyloid nematodes of equids. Infection invariably occurs through inadvertent ingestion, whether while grazing or via oral contact with elements of the environment.

Apparently, horses never develop absolute immunity to strongyloids, so these are often the sole nematode parasites recovered from well-managed, mature equids. The Strongyloidea of horses are comprised of two distinct subfamilies, the Strongylinae and the Cyathostominae.

Strongylinae (large strongyles)

Members of the subclass Strongylinae tend to be larger, on average, than most genera that comprise the Cyathostominae. In addition, Strongylinae have large buccal capsules, adapted for attachment to, and even ingestion of, the gut mucosa. The larval stages of at least one strongylin genus undergo extensive, albeit stereotypic, migration within the host prior to returning to the gut to mature and begin reproduction.

Strongylus vulgaris

Strongylus vulgaris is widely acknowledged as the single most pathogenic nematode parasite of horses. Adult worms measure about 1.5–2.5 cm in length and the females are larger than the males. Adults are usually found attached to the mucosa of the cecum and the ventral colon (Figure 1.2). After ingestion from the environment, third stage larvae invade the mucosa of the distal small intestine, cecum, and colon. Here, they molt to the fourth stage (L_4) before penetrating local

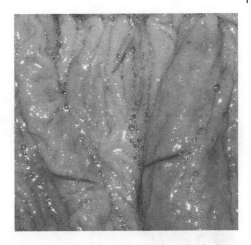

Figure 1.2 Adult *Strongylus vulgaris* attached to the cecal mucosa. (*Source*: Photograph courtesy of Dr. Tetiana Kuzmina).

arterioles and migrating proximally beneath the intimal layer of local blood vessels. Migrating *S. vulgaris* L_4s leave subintimal tracts in their wake and congregate near the root of the cranial mesenteric artery. A portion of the infecting larvae may continue to migrate, even to the root of the aorta near the left ventricle. Migrating L_4s have been found in numerous vessels arising from the aorta, including the celiac artery, the renal arteries, and external and internal iliac arteries. The pathologic characteristics and consequences of these arterial lesions will be discussed in Chapter 2.

Larvae reach the cranial mesenteric artery about two weeks post-infection. Here, they reside for about four months before returning to the large intestine. The final molt to the L_5 stage occurs about 90 days after infection, while larvae are still present in the artery. These L_5s (essentially young adults) characteristically retain their L_4 cuticle and thus appear with a double-layered cuticle just like the infective L_3 (Figure 1.3). Beginning approximately 120 days after infection, young adults migrate within the blood stream to the large intestine, where they are found within pea-sized nodules in the

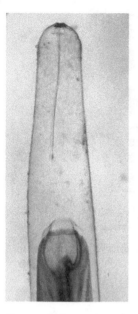

Figure 1.3 *Strongylus vulgaris* L_5 pre-adult collected from the cranial mesenteric artery. Note that this specimen characteristically has retained its L_4 cuticle.

submucosa of the ventral colon and cecum. Adult worms eventually emerge from these nodules and mature in the intestinal lumen for an additional 6 weeks. Females begin to lay eggs from 5.5 to 7 months after infection (Ogbourne and Duncan, 1985).

Strongylus edentatus
Strongylus edentatus is a larger worm than *S. vulgaris*, measuring about 2.5–4.5 cm in length, and apparently is also more prevalent. Adults are usually attached to the mucosa of the base of the cecum and the proximal ventral colon. The larvae undergo a complex and fascinating migratory route. Following ingestion of infective L_3 stages from the environment, larvae are carried by the portal system to the liver, where they molt to the fourth stage. Following migration within the parenchyma, larvae leave the liver via the hepatorenal ligament and migrate beneath the peritoneum to various locations in the flanks and ventral abdominal wall (hence, the common term, "flank worm"). Larvae are also commonly found in the perirenal fat. The majority of larvae are found on the right side of the body (*i.e.*, in the right ventral abdominal wall and around the right kidney), probably because the hepatorenal ligament attaches on the right side of the ventral midline (see Chapter 2).

The final molt to the fifth stage occurs within retroperitoneal nodules about four months post-infection. Young adults migrate back to the large intestinal walls (primarily the ventral colon), where purulent nodules form and eventually rupture to release adult worms into the lumen. Altogether, this extensive migration results in a prepatent period of up to one year (McCraw and Slocombe, 1978).

Strongylus equinus
Strongylus equinus is another large strongyle with a prolonged life cycle and a prepatent period of 8–9 months from infection to egg production. The adult worms are of about the same size as *S. edentatus*. Larvae molt to the L_4 stage upon invading the mucosa of the caecum and colon. They then migrate across the abdominal cavity and through the pancreas to finally reach the liver, where they wander for several weeks. On the way back to the large intestine, larvae again migrate through the pancreas and large L_4s and L_5s can be found free in the peritoneal cavity (McCraw and Slocombe, 1984). The third stage larvae of *S. equinus* are very distinctive in coproculture. This nematode species has become exceedingly rare in domestic herds and is not detected in managed and regularly dewormed horses. *S. equinus* can be highly prevalent and abundant in feral horses, however, and has been reported in prevalence surveys of working equids in South America (Kyvsgaard *et al.*, 2011).

Strongylus asini

Strongylus asini is a common internal parasite of zebras and donkeys in Africa. It resembles *S. vulgaris* in many ways but genetically is more closely related to *S. edentatus* and *S. equinus* (Hung *et al.*, 1996). Adults occur in the cecum and colon, but larvae are found attached to the lining of hepatic and portal veins (Malan *et al.*, 1982). Fourth stage larvae migrate within the liver and hepatic cysts are reportedly found in zebras.

Triodontophorus spp.

Although they are technically "large strongyles", the several species of *Triodontophorus* are non-migratory. The larvae encyst within the lining of the large intestine and eventually emerge to become adults. The prepatent period is thought to be approximately 2–3 months (Round, 1969). *Triodontophorus brevicauda* and *T. serratus* are probably the most prevalent species of large strongyles in managed horses, presumably because of a shorter life cycle than *Strongylus* species. One study of naturally infected horses found that the presence of *Triodontophorus* larvae in coproculture was independent of the presence of *Strongylus* spp. (Cao, Vidyashankar, and Nielsen, 2013). This finding was attributed to a shorter life cycle, which is more similar in duration to that of cyathostomins.

Triodontophorus females apparently produce eggs that are significantly larger than those of the other strongylin and cyathostomin genera (Figure 1.4).

Other strongylinae

Craterostomum acuticaudatum, Oesophagodontus robustus, and Bidentostomum ivaschkini

These species have non-migratory life cycles and are only classified as Strongylinae on the basis of their large buccal capsules (see Table 1.1). The larvae derived by coproculture can be differentiated, but as the species prevalences are so

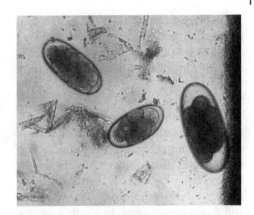

Figure 1.4 Most strongyle eggs are relatively uniform in size and shape. One exception is the eggs of *Triodontophorus* spp. (right), which are about twice the size of a typical strongyle egg. (*Source*: Photograph courtesy of Tina Roust and Maria Rhod).

Table 1.1 Examples of predilection sites of common cyathostomin species. Information from Tolliver (2000).

Cecum

Coronocyclus coronatus

Cyathostomum alveatum

Cylicocyclus elongatus

Cylicostephanus calicatus

Petrovinema poculatum

Ventral colon

Coronocyclus labiatus, Cor. labratus,

Cyathostomum catinatum, Cya. pateratum (also dorsal colon), *Cya. tetracanthum,*

Cylicocyclus auriculatus, Cyc. brevicapsulatus, Cyc. radiatus, Cyc. leptostomum Cyc. nassatus, Cyc. ashworthi, Cyc. ultrajectinus (also dorsal colon)

Cylicodontophorus bicoronatus

Cylicostephanus asymetricus, Cys. minutus

Dorsal colon

Cyathostomum pateratum (also ventral colon)

Cylicocyclus insigne, Cyc. ultrajectinus (also ventral colon)

Cylicostephanus goldi, Cys. longibursatus

Parapoteriostomum euproctus, Par. mettami

Poteriostomum imparidentum, Pot. ratzii

low, larvae are more likely to be mistaken for similar, but more common, genera. None of these species has been associated with any distinct pathology.

Cyathostominae

The Cyathostomins (also known as small strongyles, cyathostomes, or trichonemes) comprise numerous genera, including *Cylicocyclus, Cyathostomum, Cylicostephanus, Coronocyclus, Cylicodontophorus, Gyalocephalus, Poteriostomum, Petrovinema,* and *Parapoteriostomum* in North America and world-wide. Lesser-known genera, such as *Hsiungia, Tridentoinfundibulum, Skrjabinodentus, Caballonema,* and *Cylindropharynx,* have been recovered from indigenous equids in Africa and Asia (Lichtenfels, Kharchenko, and Dvojnos, 2008). The majority (>80%) of cyathostomins recovered from horses belong to just a handful of species: *Cylicocyclus nassatus, Cylicostephanus (Cys.) minutus, Cys. longibursatus, Cyathostomum catinatum,* and *Cys. calicatus* (Reinemeyer, Prado, and Nielsen, 2015) (Figure 1.5). The common term "small redworms" is misleading as adult cyathostomins are all pale white in appearance. The L_4 and early L_5 stages of *Cylicocyclus insigne* are the only cyathostomin specimens that appear red in color. *C. insigne* is a relatively large species, however, so these L_4s are easily visible in a fresh fecal sample or on a rectal palpation sleeve.

The basic life cycle of all cyathostomins is virtually identical, with development to the infective third stage in the environment. Once ingested by a horse, however, L_3 cyathostomins do not migrate systemically. (In this handbook, migration is consistently defined as leaving one organ and entering another.) Rather, incoming larvae invade the mucosa or submucosa of the cecum and ventral colon, or, to a lesser extent, the dorsal colon. Cyathostomins never encyst in the lining of the descending colon or rectum. Some species apparently invade no deeper than the mucosa,

whereas others encyst within the submucosa. In addition, species may prefer certain alimentary organs or even sites within an organ for encystment.

Cyathostomins first invade the large intestinal lining as early third stage larvae (EL_3). These are basically infective larvae that have shed their protective integument. Early L_3s are very small (<1 mm) and most genera contain only eight intestinal epithelial cells. Soon after they enter the mucosa, a fibrous capsule of host origin forms around the EL_3, and from this stage forward, these tissue larvae are referred to as "encysted" (see Chapter 2). The EL_3 is transient if the worm progresses steadily through all the larval stages to adulthood. Alternatively, individual worms may undergo arrested development and persist as EL_3s for more than a year or two.

With progressive development, the EL_3 molts into a late L_3 stage (LL_3), which is significantly larger, features a tubular buccal cavity, and has more than eight intestinal cells. The LL_3 remains within the cyst and ultimately molts into an L_4 stage, which has a distinct, goblet-shaped buccal capsule. The L_4 grows within the cyst, and eventually the cyst wall ruptures and the L_4 enters the lumen of the large intestine. This stage of emergence is also termed "excystment", which is the chief pathologic event during the cyathostomin life cycle (Chapter 2).

Within the lumen of the large intestine, an L_4 grows in size and eventually molts into the L_5 stage. Fifth stage larvae (L_5s) are basically prepubertal, non-reproductive teenagers; the transition from L_5 to adult is a gradual one, involving only maturation of the reproductive organs and an increase in body size. The L_5 develops within the sheath of the L_4 stage and individual worms that are beginning the penultimate stage of development will exhibit the buccal capsule and other cephalic features of the adult, positioned

(A)

(B)

(C)

(D)

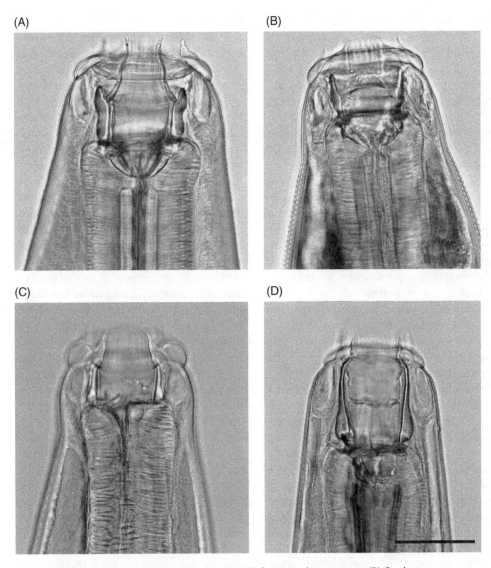

Figure 1.5 Common adult cyathostomin species. (A) *Coronocyclus coronatus*, (B) *Cyathostomum catinatum*, (C) *Cylicocyclus leptostomum*, and (D) *Petrovinema poculatum*. Size bar = 50 μm. (*Source*: Photograph courtesy of Jennifer L. Bellaw).

just beneath the remnants of the L_4 stage, which are about to be shed and discarded.

In addition to the larval stages, adult cyathostomins also exhibit distinct site preferences (Table 1.1). Although it is not unusual for each organ of the large intestine to harbor at least some specimens of any species, the majority of individuals of any species are usually recovered either

from the cecum, ventral colon, or dorsal colon. No species occupies the descending colon or rectum as a preferred niche, so specimens recovered from those locations are considered to be exiting the host.

Female cyathostomins can begin to lay eggs as soon as 5 weeks after infection (Round, 1969), but due to arrested development, some may not complete maturation until more than two years after initial ingestion by the host (Gibson, 1953). Cyathostomins can remain in arrested development longer than any other nematode group and spend their entire parasitic life cycle in the alimentary tract. The reasons for this strategy are unclear, but the evolutionary advantages are obvious. If climatic conditions did not permit prolonged environmental survival of infective stages, it would be very beneficial for the parasite if the host could carry new sources of contamination and infection wherever it went. Similarly, the same strategy would be useful if nomadic horses returned to grazing areas after intervals longer than the maximum persistence of infective stages in the environment.

Encysted cyathostomin larvae are not 100% susceptible to any known anthelmintic regimen. For this reason, it is impossible to clear a horse of all its cyathostomins. If a horse were dewormed heroically and then transferred to a sterile environment with no hope of fecal/oral reinfection, that animal would eventually begin to pass strongyle eggs again at some point in the future. As demonstrated by Smith (1976a, 1976b), if the horse were held in such an environment for a prolonged period and dewormed repeatedly, it may require more than 2 years before the sources of such episodic contamination would be permanently exhausted.

The duration of survival of adult cyathostomins has not been determined with certainty, but is thought to be on the order of three to four months.

Ascaridoidea

The superfamily Ascaridoidea is comprised of very large, stout nematodes with three prominent lips surrounding the oral opening. Some ascarid species have the most complicated life cycles of any nematode of veterinary importance, but the ascarid of horses has the simplest of all.

Parascaris spp.

Few veterinarians are aware that two species of *Parascaris* have been reported to infect horses. *Parascaris univalens* is described as a cryptic equine ascarid species that appears morphologically identical to the better-known *P. equorum*. Characteristically, specimens of *P. univalens* have only one pair of chromosomes, whereas *P. equorum* has two pairs. To date, karyotyping remains the only established technique for differentiating these two species. Both species had been described by the late 1800s, and it is an interesting item of biological trivia that the phenomenon of mitosis was first observed in the eggs of *P. univalens*. For unknown reasons, *P. univalens* has faded into obscurity, and it is rarely mentioned in veterinary textbooks. However, cell biologists and cytogeneticists have used the parasite for decades as a model for studying chromatin diminution, whereby the parasite eliminates a large proportion of its DNA during the first mitotic cell cycle (Muller and Tobler, 2000).

Contrary to prevailing wisdom, available evidence suggests that *P. equorum* may be very rare and that *P. univalens* is the more common species of equine ascarid. One study performed in Italy in the late 1970s identified over 2000 worm specimens to species level and found over 90% to be *P. univalens*, with the remainder either *P. equorum* or hybrids (Bullini *et al.*, 1978). A more recent karyotyping study performed in central Kentucky identified 30 worm specimens and 17 of 25 egg isolates to be *P. univalens*, while *P. equorum* was not identified (Nielsen *et al.*, 2014). A study of the population structure among about 200 equine ascarid parasite specimens collected in Sweden, Norway, Germany, Iceland, Brazil, and USA concluded that all specimens were genetically homogenous, and thus essentially the same species (Tyden *et al.* 2013). One isolate examined in this study was collected from a parasitology research population and subsequently identified as *P. univalens* by karyotyping. This strongly suggests that all 200 specimens from six different countries on three continents were indeed *P. univalens*. It remains possible that *P. equorum* still occurs in certain equid populations, but these need to be identified and characterized. The practical implications of these findings are currently unknown, but they may be limited to just substituting one name with another. For now, the most appropriate nomenclature to be applied for equine ascarids is "*Parascaris* spp.", unless karyotyping has been carried out to identify the specimens to species level.

Parascaris spp. is the largest intestinal nematode parasite of horses, and mature females can reach 50 cm × 1–2 cm in size (Figure 1.6) and produce approximately 200,000 eggs per day. As adults, equine ascarids reside in the small intestine, with small numbers occasionally recovered from the stomach or cecum. Females lay distinctive eggs that are passed in the feces. Under favorable environmental

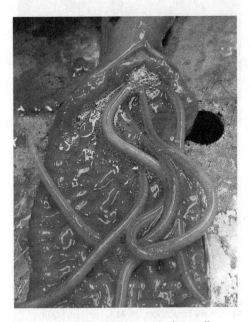

Figure 1.6 Adult *Parascaris* spp. in the small intestine of a weanling. (*Source*: Photograph courtesy of Dr. Tetiana Kuzmina).

conditions, eggs can become infective within 2 weeks. The infective stage is a larvated egg containing a coiled, third stage larva.

Horses are infected by ingesting infective ascarid eggs from the environment. The eggs are covered by a sticky, protein coating, which enables them to adhere to vertical surfaces and even to the haircoat or udder of a mare. Foals and weanlings are most commonly infected by ascarids; and transmission is greatly assisted by the tendency of juvenile horses to investigate their environments orally. Interestingly, up to 10% of ascarid eggs appearing in equine feces lack their protein coating (Donoghue *et al.*, 2015). It remains unknown whether these decorticated eggs are equally viable and able to develop into the infective stage in the environment.

When a larvated ascarid egg is ingested from the environment, the egg loses its protective coating after passing through sequential acidic and basic conditions in the stomach and small intestine, respectively. A larva emerges from the egg shell in the small intestine and penetrates the gut lining. Migrating larvae enter the lymphatics or venules draining the small intestine and are carried passively to the liver. After infection, most larvae are found in the liver within 2 to 7 days post-infection. Larvae migrate within the hepatic parenchyma, which may result in inflammatory lesions and fibrous migratory tracts. Focal, white, fibrotic lesions are often seen just below the capsule of the liver, equivalent to the condition caused in swine by migrating *Ascaris suum* (see Chapter 2).

Migrating third stage larvae are found in the lungs, beginning about two weeks after infection. Here, they exit the pulmonary venules and capillaries, and rupture alveolar membranes to enter the airways. Migrating ascarid larvae usually reside within the lungs for about two weeks. Eventually, the larvae migrate proximally in the pulmonary tree or are coughed up into the pharynx. Regardless of the mechanism, they are swallowed and return to the stomach and small intestine within 4 weeks post-infection. Once in the small intestine, the worms grow progressively, and eggs appear in the feces from 90 to 110 days post-infection (Lyons, Drudge, and Tolliver, 1976).

Adult ascarids continue to grow and may persist within the gut for several months. Ultimately, the majority of horses develop very strong immunity to *Parascaris* and egg shedding eventually ceases, even without benefit of anthelmintic treatment (Donoghue *et al.*, 2015; Fabiani, Lyons, and Nielsen, 2016). Because of this effective immunity, ascarid infections are commonly observed in sucklings, weanlings, and yearlings, but are seen only occasionally in horses older than approximately 18 months of age (Fabiani, Lyons, and Nielsen, 2016).

Recent investigations in populations of untreated foals have identified a biphasic occurrence of *Parascaris* spp. (Donoghue *et al.*, 2015; Fabiani, Lyons, and Nielsen, 2016). Adult ascarid burdens reach their peak at 4–5 months of age, as reflected by high ascarid egg counts. After this peak, the adult burdens are eliminated, but a smaller, second wave of infection can be observed at 8–10 months of age. This second infection appears to be short-lived and the adult worms are soon eliminated.

In recent years, many practitioners have observed patent ascarid infections in mature horses, and some individual adult horses resume egg-shedding repeatedly after apparently effective anthelmintic treatments. At present, it is unknown whether these recurrent infections are associated with unique immune deficiencies or with isolates of *Parascaris* that do not elicit a typical immune response, or if they merely reflect increased use of fecal egg counts to monitor horse populations.

Oxyuroidea

The Oxyuroidea, or pinworms, comprise a superfamily of nematodes that reside in a unique niche, the posterior alimentary tract. In addition to equids, other host species for pinworms include humans, rodents, primates, and sheep. The oxyuroids exhibit a unique biological adaptation in that the females do not shed eggs into the feces. Rather, they protrude from the anus and deposit eggs in a sticky film in the perineal area (Figure 1.7). The warm, moist conditions in this microhabitat likely assist in larval development. Ultimately, the dried, proteinaceous film flakes off and eggs are dropped randomly into the environment, where they may persist for several months.

Another curious piece of trivia about pinworm parasites is that their mode of reproduction is unique among nematodes. Males are derived from unfertilized

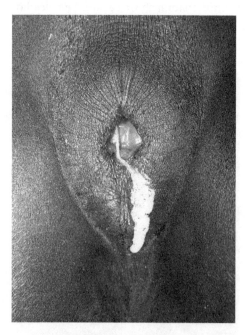

Figure 1.7 Female *Oxyuris equi* laying eggs in the perianal area. (*Source*: Reprinted from Equine Veterinary Education, 28, M.K. Nielsen, Equine tapeworm infections: Disease, diagnosis and control, pp. 388–395, Copyright (2016) with permission from EVJ Ltd, Wiley).

eggs and are thus haploid, whereas females derive from fertilized eggs and are diploid. This mode of reproduction has been termed haplodiploidy (Adamson, 1994). It is believed that this is a strategy for parasite propagation. In the absence of males, new males will automatically arise from unfertilized eggs.

Oxyuris equi

Oxyuris is the common pinworm of horses. Adult females are white, moderate in size (5–8 cm × 5 mm), and have a sharply pointed tail – thus providing the common name for this group. Males are fewer in number and only approximately one-third the size of the adult females. Adult pinworms reside in the dorsal colon, and only females can be observed commuting through the rectum to the maternity ward (Reinemeyer and Nielsen, 2014).

Female pinworms may be seen protruding from the anus, but are also observed in fresh feces or adhering to a palpation sleeve following a rectal examination. It is believed that female worms die quickly after depositing their eggs.

The larvated eggs are deposited in sheets of a sticky film, which is similar in composition to dried egg albumin. Eggs are ingested from the environment, in much the same fashion as those of *Parascaris* spp. Third stage larvae emerge from eggs in the small intestine and reportedly develop within the mucosa of the cecum and colon. As pinworms approach adulthood, they relocate to the dorsal colon. Adults do not attach to the gut wall and have negligible pathogenicity.

Probstmayria vivipara

Probstmayria is a lesser-known and extremely small pinworm that is occasionally recovered from horses. These worms are nearly invisible to the naked eye, but might be observed during microscopic examination of fresh colonic contents. This pinworm is not known to cause any distinct clinical signs. *Probstmayria's* reproductive behavior is rare among parasitic nematodes; it is viviparous and can complete its entire life cycle without leaving the host. For this reason, infections often comprise massive numbers of worms, but, again, they have no known clinical impact.

Rhabditoidea

The rhabditoid nematodes are all fairly primitive and exhibit unique life cycle adaptations such as free-living generations and an apparent absence of parasitic males.

Strongyloides westeri

Strongyloides westeri is a small nematode (6–9 mm) that parasitizes the small intestine of suckling foals. Females (parasitic males are unknown) are embedded within the mucosa at the base of the villi (Figure 1.8) and produce small (50 μm × 40 μm), thin-shelled, round to slightly elliptical eggs already containing a larva (Figure 1.9). Patent infections are

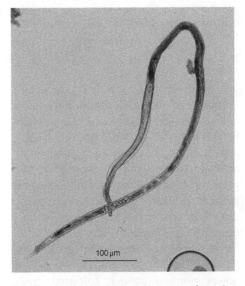

Figure 1.8 Female *Strongyloides westeri* from the small intestinal mucosa. Only females are parasitic. (*Source*: Photograph courtesy of Faith Miller).

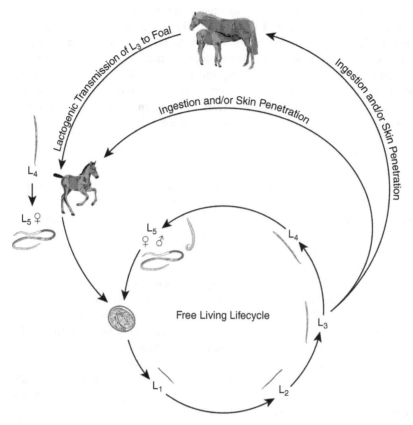

Figure 1.9 The life cycle of *Strongyloides westeri*. This parasite is capable of completing the entire cycle in the environment without entering a host. Horses can get infected by three different routes of transmission; oral ingestion of L_3 larvae, skin penetration by L_3 larvae, or lactogenic transmission of L_3s from mares to foals. Note that only the female parasites are parasitic. (*Source*: Graphics courtesy of Jamie K. Norris).

primarily seen in foals because strong immunity to *Strongyloides* develops fairly quickly, but older horses are occasionally found infected as well. Larvated eggs appearing in the feces of a yearling or older horse invariably are those of strongyles rather than *Strongyloides*. Eggs pass in the feces and L_1 larvae which emerge in the environment can follow various patterns of development (Figure 1.9). Some larvae become free-living males or females. The larvae of veterinary concern, however, are those that halt their free-living development as third stage larvae, and are restricted to a parasitic existence.

Foals can be infected with *Strongyloides* by one of three possible routes: skin penetration by third stage larvae, ingestion of third stage larvae from a contaminated environment, or lactogenic transmission from the mare. The latter route is possible because *Strongyloides* larvae do not become established in the alimentary tract of immune, adult horses. Rather, they are distributed to various somatic tissues, where they may reside for years. In mares, the hormones of pregnancy and lactation presumably stimulate the somatic larvae to resume migration and travel to the mammary glands. From this location, they are present in mare's milk from the fourth day post-partum and are ingested by suckling foals (Lyons, Drudge, and Tolliver, 1973). Numbers of larvae in the milk peak at about 10–12 days post-partum, but larvae have been recovered from milk samples up to 47 days after birth. The highest concentrations of larvae have been recovered from samples collected in the morning (Lyons, Drudge, and Tolliver, 1973).

The extent to which these lactogenic larvae undergo pulmonary migration once they reach the foal remains unclear. Available evidence suggests that lactogenically acquired larvae are quicker to develop into patent infections in foals compared with infective larvae ingested orally from the environment (Lyons, Drudge, and Tolliver, 1973). One possible explanation is that lactogenic larvae do not have a tissue migration stage within the foals. Larvae acquired via the transcutaneous route, however, do migrate through the lungs before establishing in the small intestine.

Most *S. westeri* infections in foals are asymptomatic, but symptomatic infections will be described in Chapter 2.

Halicephalobus deletrix

Halicephalobus (syn: *Micronema*) is a free-living rhabditoid nematode that occasionally takes up residence within living tissues. It usually gains entry to the mammalian body through grossly contaminated lacerations or possibly through mucous membranes. *Halicephalobus* causes granulomatous lesions and is locally or systemically invasive. Spontaneous infections are seen occasionally in horses and generally involve cephalic tissues (gingiva and underlying bone, sinuses, brain) or well-vascularized organs such as the kidney (Ferguson *et al.*, 2011). Recent observations have provided evidence of a hematogenous spread of this parasite to these distant sites (Henneke *et al.*, 2014). Human infections have been reported, but generally are subsequent to severe tissue damage and gross contamination with manure or soil.

Atypically for most parasitic nematodes, adult *Halicephalobus* reproduce within the host, resulting in superinfections with adults and larvae in all stages of development.

Spiruroidea

All spiruroid nematodes require an arthropod intermediate host for transmission to a vertebrate vector. The spiruroids affecting horses occur either as adults in stereotypic locations or as larvae in a variety of aberrant tissues.

Habronema muscae

Habronema muscae are approximately 1 to 2.5 cm in length and occur in the stomach of equids. They produce very tiny ($16\,\mu m \times 45\,\mu m$), thin-shelled, larvated eggs that are passed in the feces. In the environment, larvae emerge and are ingested by adult dipterans (*e.g.*, *Musca domestica*) or are swallowed by feeding maggots. Infection is completed via ingestion of dead flies in feed stuffs or water. Alternatively, infective *Habronema* larvae may travel to the mouth parts of living flies and be deposited in wounds or at mucocutaneous junctions during feeding activities.

Within the stomach, the parasites become adults in about eight weeks. Adult *Habronema* are found in close contact with the gastric mucosa, but they cause no clinical problems. The larvae deposited in wounds or at mucocutaneous junctions, however, can result in proliferative, ulcerated lesions that tend to increase in size throughout the fly season (see Chapter 2).

Habronema microstoma

Habronema microstoma is a less common species in this superfamily that uses stable flies (*Stomoxys calcitrans*) as intermediate hosts. There are no major differences in the biology or pathogenicity of the two *Habronema* species.

Draschia megastoma

The life cycle of *Draschia megastoma* is virtually identical to that of the *Habronema* spp. and the house fly (*Musca domestica*) is the preferred intermediate host. The major biological difference is that adult specimens of *Draschia* are found in large (5 cm × 5 cm), tumor-like, fibrous masses that are usually located near the *margo plicatus* of the stomach. The *margo* is the junction of the glandular and non-glandular gastric epithelium of equids. *Draschia* adults and associated lesions were observed in 22 of 55 horses necropsied in 1984 (Reinemeyer *et al.*, 1984). However, *D. megastoma* apparently has become quite rare because none of the authors has seen a single gastric lesion in hundreds of horses necropsied since ~1985.

Thelazia lacrymalis

Horses are the definitive hosts of one species of *Thelazia*, or eye worms. As adults, *Thelazia* are found within the conjunctival *cul de sac* or beneath the nictitating membrane. Adult females produce larvae, which are present in the tear film of an infected eye. The usual intermediate host is the house fly, *Musca domestica*, or face fly, *Musca autumnalis*. Apparently, flies feeding on ocular discharges ingest larvae, which then develop to the infective stage within the body of the fly. Another horse is infected when the vector fly returns to feed on its lacrimal secretions. Infective stages leave the mouth parts of the fly, enter the conjunctival sac of the horse, and initiate a new infection.

Eye worms are thought to be relatively innocuous.

Filarioidea

The filarioidea comprise a superfamily of long, thin nematodes that often reside in organs with no direct connection to the external environment. Therefore, these worms are challenged with disseminating their reproductive products away from the host so they can undergo the development necessary to infect a new generation of hosts. Filarioids accomplish this goal by producing small, motile, reproductive stages known as microfilariae. Microfilariae circulate in the blood or lymph, or migrate to the skin. From these locations, they are ingested by arthropod intermediate hosts which feed on the tissues or secretions of live horses.

Onchocerca

Onchocerca cervicalis and *O. gutturosa* adults are sometimes referred to as "neck threadworms" because they are found deep in the connective tissues of the nuchal ligament. Adults of *O. reticulata* reside in connective tissues in the distal limbs. Microfilariae are produced by female worms, and they enter the circulatory system and travel to the dermis and epidermis. Here, they are ingested by feeding *Culicoides* (midges) or *Simulium* (black flies). Microfilariae develop within the tissues of the fly, migrate to the dipteran mouth parts as infective L_3s, and reinfect another equid during subsequent feeding episodes. In the new host, infective stages migrate to the target connective tissues and begin reproducing ~6 months after inoculation. Adult worms are capable of remaining alive for several years. The prevalence of *Onchocerca* spp. is generally unknown in managed horses, but one survey in central Kentucky found that 24% of examined horses harbored adult worms (Lyons *et al.*, 2000).

Setaria equina

Setaria equina is a filarioid nematode that resides free within the abdominal cavity of equids. Although not pathogenic, it is a very prominent finding at necropsy, which is hard to disavow in the presence of lay witnesses. Microfilariae are produced within the peritoneal cavity, but enter the circulation and can be found in peripheral blood. From here, they are ingested by feeding mosquitos, and transmission is similar to that described earlier for the genus *Onchocerca*.

Parafilaria multipapillosa

Adult *Parafilaria* occur in subcutaneous and intermuscular connective tissue of horses. Nodules form in the overlying skin, and the nodules may rupture and bleed or leak tissue fluids. First stage larvae are present in the exudate from bleeding lesions and are ingested by feeding horn flies (*Hematobia irritans*). Larvae develop to the infective third stage within the fly and are transferred to horses when flies feed on lachrymal secretions or skin wounds. The larvae then migrate in the subcutaneous tissues and develop to the adult stage within a year. Eggs and microfilariae can readily be identified in smears taken from lesion exudates.

Trichostrongyloidea

Trichostrongyloids are fairly small nematodes that reside within the stomach or abomasum and small intestine of grazing animals. Most trichostrongyloids are parasites of ruminants. The free-living portions of the life cycle are virtually identical to those of the strongyloid nematodes discussed earlier.

Trichostrongylus axei

Trichostrongylus axei is the only gastrointestinal nematode that horses share with other domestic animals. This parasite occurs in the abomasum of sheep, cattle, and goats, and there is some possibility of cross-infection among the various host species.

T. axei females reside in the stomach, and produce eggs which are deposited in feces. They are fairly similar to those of the strongyloid group, but tend to be slightly smaller, more delicate, and one end of the egg is somewhat pointed. *Trichostrongylus* infection can be diagnosed readily by differential coproculture (see Chapter 9). Horses are infected by accidental ingestion of larvae during grazing. Incoming larvae invade gastric glands and develop to the adult stage, whereupon they emerge into the lumen and begin to lay eggs 3 to 4 weeks after infection.

In ruminants, *T. axei* infection is susceptible to anthelmintics of the benzimidazole and macrocyclic lactone classes; similar efficacy is likely in horses. However, a specific label claim does not exist for any equine products, due to the difficulty of demonstrating efficacy against infections of such low prevalence.

Dictyocaulus arnfieldi

Dictyocaulus arnfieldi is the lungworm of equids. Adults live in the terminal bronchioles and can be found in the major airways. Gravid females deposit eggs in bronchial secretions, which are carried proximally by the ciliary apparatus or spontaneous coughing. From the pharynx, the larvae are swallowed and then passed in the feces. Diagnosis involves using the Baermann technique to demonstrate larvae in the feces.

D. arnfieldi is considered a normal parasite of donkeys, because it reproduces readily and induces little pathogenicity. Horses, however, will rarely support an infection to the adult stage because they are not suitable definitive hosts. Infected horses usually have a history of sharing common pasture with donkeys.

Cestodes

Anoplocephalinae

Equids harbor three species of cestodes, but only one of those can be considered common. All are members of a closely related family and, like nearly all other cestodes, require an intermediate host for transmission. Unlike nematodes, equine cestodes apparently do not release individual eggs on a regular basis. Rather, terminal (gravid) proglottids probably detach and disintegrate during transit to the external environment (Figure 1.10).

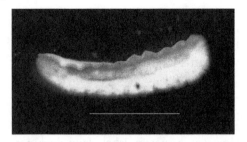

Figure 1.10 Gravid proglottid (tapeworm segment) of *Anoplocephala perfoliata*. Size bar = 1 cm. (*Source:* Photograph courtesy of Jamie K. Norris).

This results in a rather patchy distribution of cestode eggs within the fecal output of infected horses, with obvious diagnostic implications (see Chapter 9).

In the environment, cestode eggs within feces are ingested by free-living mites of the family Oribatidae, which are endemic in soils world-wide. After ingestion, an oncosphere (essentially the scolex of a future adult worm) is digested from the egg within the alimentary tract of the mite. The oncosphere migrates into the hemocoel (body cavity) of the mite and develops into an infective stage known as a cysticercoid (Figure 1.11). Cysticercoids probably remain infective for the lifespan of the mite host and it is likely that infected mites can persist in the environment for longer than a single season.

Horses are infected via inadvertent ingestion of vector mites while grazing. The cysticercoids are digested free of the mite's tissue in the horse's gastrointestinal tract and primitive scolices attach to the lining of the preferred region of gut. Adult cestodes are able to regenerate an entire organism (known as a strobila) from the attached scolex.

Anoplocephala perfoliata

Anoplocephala perfoliata is the most common cestode of equids world-wide, and has been reported from every continent except Antarctica. It is a moderately sized worm, ranging from 1 to 8 cm in length and 1 to 2 cm in width and can be identified by the presence of lappets beneath each of the four suckers on the scolex (Figure 1.12). Proglottids are very small (10–20 mm by 5 mm, but <1 mm thick) and have a yellow-grayish appearance (Figure 1.10). Unlike the cestodes of other mammalian species, it is rare to observe proglottids in the feces of horses, at least of those infected with *A. perfoliata*. *Anoplocephala* infection can be diagnosed by fecal examination, but this technique has fairly low sensitivity in horses, as discussed elsewhere (see Chapter 9).

A. perfoliata is a rare exception to the rule that all adult cestodes reside within the small intestine of their vertebrate host. Adult and developing *A. perfoliata* are mostly found attached to the lining of the cecum and the majority tend to cluster around the cecal side of the ileocecal valve. Additional masses of cestodes are sometimes observed at various locations in the cecum and individual specimens may be attached to the mucosa of the ventral colon or ileum. The longevity of individual specimens of *A. perfoliata* is unknown, but tapeworms mature and remain within the gut through the winter, to be replaced by a new burden during the grazing season.

Several studies have demonstrated a clear, seasonal pattern in the prevalence and abundance of *A. perfoliata*. In temperate climates, most patent infections are observed in the second half of the year, reflecting infections that were acquired and established over the preceding grazing season (Meana *et al.*, 2005).

Anoplocephala magna

True to its name, *A. magna* is the largest cestode occurring in equids and may achieve 80 cm in length. *A. magna* normally attaches to the mucosa in the distal small intestine and can be differentiated from *A. perfoliata* by its relative size and preferred location in the host. For definitive identification of individual specimens

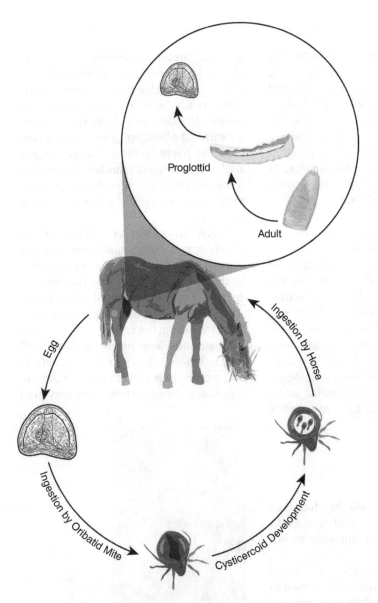

Figure 1.11 Life cycle of *Anoplocephala perfoliata*. Oribatid mites act as intermediate hosts and are ingested by horses while grazing. Proglottids are released from adult tapeworms and are subsequently disintegrated to liberate the eggs inside. (*Source*: Graphics courtesy of Jamie K. Norris).

Figure 1.12 Anterior end of an *Anoplocephala perfoliata* specimen obtained from the cecum of a horse at necropsy. This species is characterized by four suckers (arrow heads) with corresponding lappets (arrows) just beneath them. (*Source*: Photograph courtesy of Jamie K. Norris).

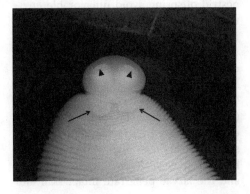

A. magna lacks the lappets described for *A. perfoliata* above. Proglottids of *A. magna* are between 2 and 5 cm wide and can sometimes be observed in the feces.

Nearly a century ago, *A. magna* was reportedly far more prevalent than *A. perfoliata*, but the relative ranking of these species has reversed over time. At the present time, *A. magna* is encountered infrequently world-wide.

Anoplocephaloides mamillana (formerly Paranoplocephala mamillana)

This is a very uncommon parasite of equids, which normally attaches to the mucosa of the proximal small intestine. It is a very tiny worm, only 6–50 mm long and 4–6 mm wide. Proglottids are similarly small, about 2 by 5 mm, but are sometimes observed motile in the feces. *A. mamillana* is little more than a biological oddity and diagnostic differential; infections are not known to have any clinical impact.

Arthropods

Only one arthropod will be discussed herein, namely members of the genus *Gasterophilus*, known commonly as bot flies.

Horse bot flies are members of a larger family, known as oestrid flies. Although the biological details and the host distributions differ markedly, all oestrid flies employ the same general strategy. Accordingly, oestrid offspring avoid unfavorable environmental conditions by passing their immature stages (termed "instars") within the body of an intended host. The oestrids of large domestic animals deposit eggs or larvae directly onto the intended host. Once the larval stage becomes active (after egg-hatching in some cases), they enter the host by specific routes. Thus, some oestrids (*e.g.*, *Hypoderma* of cattle) hatch from eggs attached to the hair coat, and the larvae penetrate intact skin and

undergo sustained systemic migrations. Others (*e.g.*, *Oestrus* of sheep) are deposited as larvae within the nares and migrate only locally and develop within the sinuses. In most cases, the larvae overwinter within the host, emigrate from the host in spring, pupate in the soil, and emerge as adults to complete another generation. Most oestrids are univoltine, meaning they propagate only a single generation per year.

Female flies of the genus *Gasterophilus* attach eggs to individual hairs of equid hosts (Figure 1.13) and larvae gain access to the oral cavity via routes that vary by species. Bot larvae generally overwinter within the equine alimentary tract, pass from the host in the feces during spring or early summer, and pupate in loose soil. Adult flies emerge from the soil one to two months later and emerge to mate and reproduce. Adult oestrids have very brief

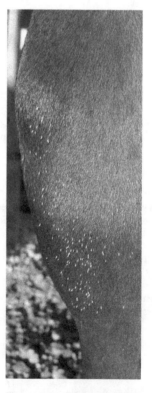

Figure 1.13 *Gasterophilus* spp. eggs attached to the haircoat of the leg.

life spans, due in part to the absence of mouthparts, which renders them incapable of ingesting nutrients.

Gasterophilus intestinalis

Gasterophilus intestinalis is the most prevalent and numerous of the bot species in domesticated horses. Female flies hover and glue individual eggs to hair shafts on the distal forelimbs and occasionally along the neck and mane. Eggs hatch in response to contact with a horse's lips (Bello, 1967), hatch immediately, and attach to the lips and tongue. Eggs that are laid on the mane are probably ingested by herd mates during mutual grooming. First instar larvae burrow into the tongue, creating small airshafts in their wake in the process. First instars are reported to remain within the tongue for up to 21 days (Cogley, Anderson, and Cogley, 1982). They subsequently migrate to the gingival pockets around the molars and premolars, where they molt to the second instar. After about 4 weeks in the oral cavity, they relocate to the stomach, where they attach to the mucosa in the non-glandular portion and develop to the third instar. *G. intestinalis* third instar larvae are about 2 cm long and 5–8 mm wide, dark brownish red in color, and have several rows of spines (Figure 1.14). Burdens of several hundred bots are common in horses, and can be visualized easily and even enumerated gastroscopically.

Gasterophilus nasalis

Female *Gasterophilus nasalis* flies deposit their eggs in the intermandibular area. The eggs hatch spontaneously and larvae crawl independently to the lips, enter the oral cavity, and develop in pockets in the tongue and around the cheek teeth. Ultimately, second instars are swallowed and continue their development in the alimentary tract. Second and third instar *G. nasalis* prefer to attach in the

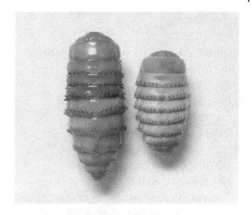

Figure 1.14 Third instars of *Gasterophilus intestinalis* (left) and *G. nasalis* (right). Note the characteristic double rows of spines on *G. intestinalis*. (*Source*: Photograph courtesy of Jennifer L. Bellaw).

ampulla of the duodenum, just a few centimeters past the pylorus.

Other *Gasterophilus* species

Other bot species that apparently do not occur in North America include *Gasterophilus inermis* and *G. hemorrhoidalis*. The latter species attaches in masses in the distal small colon and rectum of donkeys in Africa, and has been documented as a cause of rectal prolapse. Other minor species are distributed around the globe, but none has distinctive pathogenicity.

Trematodes

Trematodes are uncommon parasites of horses in most developed countries. The liver fluke, *Fasciola hepatica*, occasionally infects horses, but is seen only in areas where fascioliasis is endemic in traditional, ruminant hosts. Horses with liver fluke infections inevitably have been pastured where microclimates favor the development of molluscan intermediate hosts. Readers are referred to Nansen, Andersen, and Hesselholt (1975) for a detailed description of the life cycle and clinical features of equine *Fasciola* infection.

References

Adamson, M. (1994) Evolutionary patterns in life histories of Oxyurida. *Int. J. Parasitol.*, 24, 1167–1177.

Bello, T.R. (1967) *In vitro* hatching of *Gasterophilus intestinalis* larvae. *J. Parasitol.*, 53, 859–862.

Bullini, L., Nascetti, G., Ciafre, S., *et al.* (1978) Ricerche cariologiche ed elettroforetiche su *Parascaris univalens* e *Parascaris equorum. Acc. Naz. Lincei Rend. Cl. Sc. Fis. Mat. Nat.*, 65, 151–156.

Cao, X., Vidyashankar, A.N., and Nielsen, M.K. (2013) Association between large strongyle genera in larval cultures – using rare-event Poisson regression. *Parasitology*, 140, 1246–1251.

Cogley, T.P., Anderson, J.R., and Cogley, L.J. (1982) Migration of *Gasterophilus intestinalis* larvae (Diptera: Gasterophilidae) in the equine oral cavity. *Int. J. Parasitol.*, 12, 473–480.

Donoghue, E.M., Lyons, E.T., Bellaw, J.L., and Nielsen, M.K. (2015) Biphasic appearance of corticated and decorticated ascarid egg shedding in untreated horse foals. *Vet. Parasitol.*, 214, 114–117.

Fabiani, J.V., Lyons, E.T., and Nielsen, M.K. (2016) Dynamics of *Parascaris* and *Strongylus* spp. parasites in untreated juvenile horses. *Vet. Parasitol.*, 30, 62–66.

Ferguson, R., van Dreumel, T., Keystone, J.S., *et al.* (2008) Unsuccessful treatment of a horse with mandibular granulomatous osteomyelitis due to *Halicephalobus gingivalis. Can. Vet. J.*, 49, 1099–1103.

Gibson, T.E. (1953) The effect of repeated anthelmintic treatment with phenothiazine on fecal egg counts of housed horses, with some observations on the life cycle of *Trichonema* spp. in the horse. *J. Helminthol.*, 27, 29–40.

Henneke, C., Jespersen, A., Jacobsen, S., *et al.* (2014) The distribution pattern of *Halicephalobus gingivalis* in a horse is suggestive of a haematogenous spread of the nematode. *Acta Vet. Scand.*, 56, 56.

Hung, G.C., Jacobs, D.E., Krecek, R.C., *et al.* (1996) *Strongylus asini* (Nematoda: Strongyloidea): Genetic relationships with other *Strongylus* species determined by ribosomal DNA. *Int. J. Parasitol.*, 26, 1408–1411.

Kyvsgaard, N.C., Lindbom, J., Andreasen, L.L., *et al.* 2011. Prevalence and anthelmintic control of strongyles in working horses in Nicaragua. *Vet. Parasitol.*, 181, 248–254.

Lichtenfels, J.R., Kharchenko, V.A., and Dvojnos, G.M. (2008) Illustrated identification keys to strongylid parasites (Strongylidae: Nematoda) of horses, zebras and asses (Equidae). *Vet. Parasitol.*, 156, 4–161.

Lyons, E.T., Drudge, J.H., and Tolliver, S.C. (1973) Life-cycle of *Strongyloides westeri* in equine. *J. Parasitol.* 59, 780–787.

Lyons, E.T., Drudge, J.H., and Tolliver, S.C. (1976) Studies on the development and chemotherapy of larvae of *Parascaris equorum* (Nematoda: Ascaridoidea) in experimental and naturally infected foals. *J. Parasitol.*, 62, 453–459.

Lyons, E.T., Swerczek, T.W., Tolliver, S.C., *et al.* 2000. Prevalence of selected species of internal parasites in equids at necropsy in central Kentucky (1995–1999). *Vet. Parasitol.*, 92, 51–62.

Malan, F.S., Vos, V., de Reinecke, R.K., Pletcher, J.M. (1982) Studies on *Strongylus asini*. I. Experimental infestation of equines. *Onderstepoort J. Vet. Res.*, 49, 151–153.

McCraw, B.M. and Slocombe, J.O.D. (1978) *Strongylus edentatus*: Development and lesions from ten weeks postinfection to patency. *Can. J. Comp. Med.*, 42, 340–356.

McCraw, B.M. and Slocombe, J.O.D. (1984) *Strongylus equinus*: Development and pathological effects in the equine host. *Can. J. Comp. Med.*, 49, 372–383.

Meana, A., Pato, N.F., Martin, R., *et al.* (2005) Epidemiological studies on equine cestodes in central Spain: Infection pattern and population dynamics. *Vet. Parasitol.*, 130, 233–240.

Muller, F. and Tobler, H. (2000) Chromatin diminution in the parasitic nematodes *Ascaris suum* and *Parascaris univalens. Int. J. Parasitol.*, 30, 391–399.

Nansen, P., Andersen, S., and Hesselholt, M. (1975) Experimental infection of the horse with *Fasciola hepatica. Exp. Parasitol.*, 37, 15–19.

Nielsen, M.K., Wang, J., Davis, R., *et al.* (2014) *Parascaris univalens* – a victim of large-scale misidentification? *Parasitol. Res.*, 113, 4485–4490.

Ogbourne, C.P. and Duncan, J.L. (1985) *Strongylus vulgaris* in the horse: its biology and importance. Commonwealth Institute of Parasitology, Commonwealth Institute of Helminthology, no. 9.

Reinemeyer, C.R. and Nielsen, M.K. (2014) Review of the biology and control of *Oxyuris equi. Equine Vet. Educ.*, 26, 584–591.

Reinemeyer, C.R., Prado, J.C., and Nielsen, M.K. (2015) Comparison of the larvicidal efficacies of moxidectin or a five-day regimen of fenbendazole in horses harbouring cyathostomin populations resistant to the adulticidal dosage of fenbendazole. *Vet. Parasitol.*, 214, 100–107.

Reinemeyer, C.R., Smith, S.A., Gabel, A.A., and Herd, R.P. (1984) The prevalence and intensity of internal parasites of horses in the U.S.A. *Vet. Parasitol.*, 15, 75–83.

Round, M.C. (1969) The prepatent period of some horse nematodes determined by experimental infection. *J. Helminthol.*, 43, 185–192.

Smith, H.J. (1976a) Strongyle infections in ponies. I. Response to intermittent thiabendazole treatments. *Can. J. Comp. Med.*, 40, 327–333.

Smith, H.J. (1976b) Strongyle infections in ponies. II. Reinfection of treated animals. *Can. J. Comp. Med.*, 40, 334–340.

Tolliver, S.C. (2000) A practical method of identification of the North American Cyathostomes (small strongyles) in equids in Kentucky. Kentucky Agricultural Experiment Station, Department of Veterinary Science, University of Kentucky, USA.

Tyden, E., Morrison, D.A., Engstrom, A., *et al.* (2013) Population genetics of *Parascaris equorum* based on whole genome DNA fingerprinting. *Infect. Genet. Evol.*, 13, 236–241.

2

Pathology of Parasitism and Impact on Performance

Conventional wisdom maintains that parasitic organisms are inherently harmful and the purported consequences of parasitism are legion (weight loss, diarrhea, anemia, hypoproteinemia, inflammation, etc.). However, there is a great distinction between parasitic infection (*i.e.*, their mere presence) and parasitic disease. All humans harbor *Escherichia coli* and *Staphylococcus aureus*, but these unbidden guests are tolerated as normal host flora until something upsets the balance. Yet somehow, the distinction between infection and disease seems much easier to ignore when the putative pathogen is grossly visible.

Unlike viral, bacterial, and fungal pathogens, nematode parasites (with rare exceptions) cannot amplify their numbers within the host. Consequently, the designation of disease along the continuum of parasitic infection depends on the magnitude of exposure, as well as the host's reaction (or inability to react) to the parasites and the changes they induce. Clinical parasitosis could be described accurately as the culmination of thousands of microinsults.

Animals vary widely in their susceptibility to parasitic disease and certain individuals apparently experience far more damage from a standard number of parasites than a typical member of their species. In sheep and cattle parasitisms, it has been demonstrated that some elements of a host's ability to limit parasite numbers, and thus their susceptibility to disease, are determined genetically (Gasbarre, Leighton, and Davies, 1990; Davies *et al.*, 2006). This is also likely to be the case for horses. However, in addition, ancillary factors such as malnutrition, stress, immunosuppression, or concomitant illness famously predispose hosts to parasitic disease.

Parasitosis in an individual animal can develop from a variety of factors, some host and some management. When parasitic disease develops in a population of animals, however, the root cause invariably is related to management. The influence of various management practices on the size and potential damage of parasite populations is addressed in Chapter 6. The present chapter will focus on the pathogenic mechanisms specific to various helminth parasites of the horse and the potential clinical manifestations in individual animals.

Nematodes

Strongylinae (large strongyles)

In the adult stage, large strongyles are found attached to the lining of the cecum and colon. Their large buccal capsules enable them to "inhale" plugs of mucosa and to ingest nutrients in the form of blood, plasma, or mucosal cells. Although attached strongyles may cause focal inflammation and ulceration, the

Handbook of Equine Parasite Control, Second Edition. Martin K. Nielsen and Craig R. Reinemeyer.
© 2018 John Wiley & Sons, Inc. Published 2018 by John Wiley & Sons, Inc.

contribution of adult stages to strongyle disease is modest. Blood loss due to strongyle feeding is insufficient to cause clinical anemia because strongyles are rarely present in high enough numbers to reduce the packed cell volume to dangerous levels. Rather, the major pathology caused by large strongyles can be attributed to their migrating stages (Ogbourne and Duncan, 1985).

Strongylus vulgaris

The migratory pattern of *S. vulgaris* was described previously in Chapter 1. The migration of fourth stage larvae results in fibrous tracts beneath the intimal layer of the mesenteric arteries and abdominal aorta (Figure 2.1). After migrating larvae reach the cranial mesenteric artery and its major branches, they increase greatly in size and molt to the fifth stage. A smaller proportion of larvae invariably reach the celiac artery as well. The presence of L_5s is associated with severe local arteritis, fibrinous exudate, thrombi within the vessel lumen, and hypertrophy and fibrosis of the medial layer (Figure 2.2). The resulting enlargement of the root of the CMA (often termed a verminous aneurysm) is a very prominent lesion at

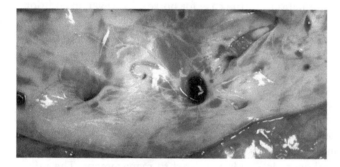

Figure 2.1 Migratory tracts caused by migrating *Strongylus vulgaris* larvae in the abdominal aorta. The two large arteries branching off in this region are the celiac artery (left) and the cranial mesenteric artery (center). L_4 and L_5 stage larvae of *S. vulgaris* can be found in both of these arteries.

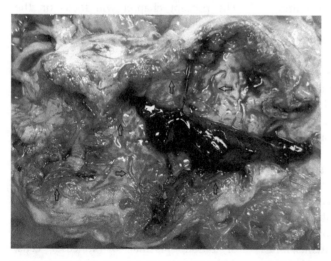

Figure 2.2 Verminous endarteritis caused by migrating *Strongylus vulgaris* larvae in the cranial mesenteric artery. The lesion is characterized by an increased diameter of the vessel, a fibrotic thickening of the arterial wall, presence of blood clots, fibrin and parasitic larvae (arrows) in the vessel lumen.

necropsy (Ogbourne and Duncan, 1985) and can sometimes be palpated per rectum in small horses.

When fifth stage larvae are ready to return to the gut, the mesenteric circulation carries them distally to the large intestinal wall. The larvae exit the terminal arterioles and form fibrous abscesses within the wall of the cecum and to a lesser extent the ventral colon. These abscesses are approximately 5 to 8 mm in diameter, thick-walled, and filled with purulent material, whether occupied by a larva or recently vacated. Interestingly, these rather prominent lesions have not been associated with any kind of clinical manifestations.

The incidence of colic has long been attributed to the prevalence of *S. vulgaris* and the associated arteritis and thromboembolism, but formal evidence for this assumed correlation is anecdotal at best. It has been established that monospecific *S. vulgaris* infections in susceptible foals can result in severe and fatal disease (Duncan and Pirie, 1975). However, despite the severity of arterial lesions, the pathophysiology of the purported colic episodes is not clear-cut. A simplistic explanation is that thrombi arise from inflammatory granulation tissue, detach from the arteritis lesions, and are then embolized distally until they reach a terminal branch sufficiently small to become occluded (Enigk, 1951). However, a postmortem survey of horses with ischemic bowel lesions failed to demonstrate emboli in the majority of cases (White, 1985). It has also been hypothesized that *S. vulgaris* larvae cause colic by interfering with local neurologic control of gut motility (Wright, 1972).

Recent work has suggested that migrating *S. vulgaris* larvae can elicit mild activation of coagulation, fibrinolysis, and inflammation (Pihl, Nielsen, and Jacobsen, 2017), but it remains unknown how this pathogenesis contributes to clinical colic. It is possible that *S. vulgaris*-associated

colic may simply be caused by the migration of L_5 larvae back to the intestine, without the presence of thromboemboli. Larvae that are unable to escape from arterioles while attempting to invade the intestinal wall may cause local endarteritis, which could occlude the vessel in question and lead to ischemia and infarction.

Recent work has illustrated that clinical cases of *S. vulgaris*-associated colic are characterized by non-strangulating intestinal infarctions (Nielsen *et al.*, 2016). While this condition can be initially painful, a majority of cases do not exhibit dramatic signs of colic, and the clinical picture is dominated by peritonitis (Pihl *et al.*, in press). If abdominocentesis is not performed by the primary attending veterinarian, diagnosis may be delayed until the case is transferred to a referral hospital. Even then, a specific cause for the peritonitis may not be identifiable without exploratory laparotomy. Infarcted areas of bowel are typically located in the cecum or the left ventral colon (Figure 2.3), and one study reported only a 10% survival rate (Pihl *et al.*, in press). Attempts to treat the condition medically were uniformly unsuccessful and all surviving cases had undergone a successful resection of the infarcted intestine.

Strongylus edentatus

Following ingestion, *S. edentatus* L_3s exsheathe in the small intestine, penetrate the gut, and migrate in the liver and retroperitoneal space. Larvae are commonly found beneath the peritoneum along the body wall or in perirenal fat deposits. Migrating larvae are grossly visible (2–3 cm in length) and embedded in discolored lesions with evidence of hemorrhage and edema (Figure 2.4). Incising the peritoneum over these lesions typically releases a large, sluggish larva. Migratory *S. edentatus* larvae have been associated with liver pathology and peritonitis (McCraw and Slocombe, 1978). The clinical impact of these migratory

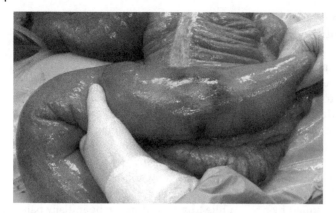

Figure 2.3 A non-strangulating infarction in the intestinal wall of the pelvic flexure of the ventral colon caused by *Strongylus vulgaris*. (*Source*: Photograph courtesy of Dr. Stine Jacobsen).

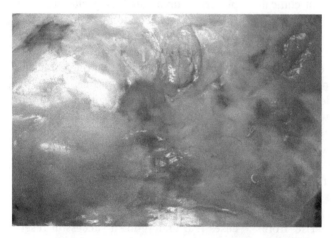

Figure 2.4 *Strongylus edentatus* larvae in the ventral abdominal wall. Larvae migrate sub- and retroperitoneally and cause local hemorrhages. Incising these lesions reveals large strongyle larvae. (*Source*: Photograph courtesy of Dr. Tetiana Kuzmina).

lesions is unknown, but they likely contribute to a general syndrome of strongylosis in heavily parasitized horses.

Mature larvae return to the ventral colon by migrating beneath the peritoneum to the adventitial layer of the large intestine, with further migration into the submucosa. Intramural abscesses develop, as for *S. vulgaris*, but they tend to be slightly larger.

Strongylus equinus

This large strongyle species has become extremely rare in managed horses, so its inclusion here is merely for the sake of completeness. *S. equinus* larvae have a distinct preference for migrating within the pancreas and in the abdominal cavity before entering the liver. Mature larvae eventually return to the gut in much the same fashion as *S. edentatus*. Pathological lesions include pancreatitis with subsequent pancreatic dysfunction, liver pathology, and peritonitis (McCraw and Slocombe, 1984).

Strongylus asini

Very little information is available about this parasite, but peritonitis has been associated with migrating *S. asini* larvae (Jaskoski and Colglazier, 1956).

Triodontophorus spp.

Although *Triodontophorus* spp. are technically large strongyles (Strongylinae), their life cycle does not include a migratory stage, so they are more similar to the cyathostomins in that regard. Adults of the two most common species, *T. serratus* and *T. brevicauda*, attach to the mucosa of the cecum and ventral colon, similar to the genus *Strongylus*. Although specimens of *Triodontophorus* are usually more numerous than *Strongylus* spp., they are substantially smaller and presumably cause little mechanical damage as adults.

One species, *T. tenuicollis*, causes pathognomonic lesions in the dorsal colon consisting of deep ulcers that are approximately 1 to 4 cm in diameter and tightly packed with dark black material. The ulcer contents separate easily from the underlying mucosa, but when the dark material is teased apart, one finds that it is comprised of tightly woven specimens of adult *T. tenuicollis*, often numbering in the dozens (Drudge, 1972). The black material around the worms may be accumulations of copulatory cement. Male nematodes secrete copulatory cement to seal the vagina of the female after mating. This reproductive strategy putatively deprives other males of the opportunity to pass on their genetic material. These "worm nests" are observed almost exclusively in horses less than 2 years of age. No specific clinical signs have been attributed to these verminous ulcers and it is unknown whether test results for fecal albumin and hemoglobin would be similar to other causes of dorsal colonic ulceration. In any case, *T. tenuicollis* ulcers remain an interesting item of trivia for pathologists.

Cyathostominae (small strongyles; Trichonemes)

Large strongyles were ubiquitous and virtually uncontrollable prior to the development of effective equine anthelmintics. In consequence, minimal, if any, pathogenicity was historically attributed to cyathostomins. However, as routine anthelmintic use eventually diminished the prevalence and importance of large strongyles, distinct syndromes of parasitic disease were recognized and ultimately attributed to small strongyles.

Cyathostomins are currently considered among the most important nematode pathogens of mature horses. This distinction was not gained by overwhelming pathogenicity, but rather was earned largely by default because: (1) large strongyles have been controlled effectively on well-managed farms, (2) other nematode pathogens (*e.g.*, *Parascaris* spp.) are controlled by immunity, so their impact is limited almost exclusively to juveniles, and (3) the remaining, prevalent parasites of adult horses (*e.g.*, bots and pinworms) are not very pathogenic. Although 50 species of cyathostomins have been described, they are traditionally regarded as a homogeneous group with similar life cycles and common modes of pathogenicity.

Our current knowledge of cyathostomin pathogenicity is fairly limited, but some general themes can be described. The pathologic events and health consequences differ with the various stages of the cyathostomin life cycle, so these will be discussed chronologically.

Mucosal invasion

Infective third stage cyathostomin larvae are ingested from the environment by grazing horses. Within the lumen of the small intestine, acid/base conditions and enzymatic activity remove the protective sheath from each larva, revealing a minute (<1 mm) organism with only eight intestinal epithelial cells and a very small oral cavity. When the exsheathed L_3s reach the cecum or ventral colon, they enter the glands of Lieberkühn and penetrate cells at the base. These glands are deformed by the presence of growing larvae, and localized hypertrophy and hyperplasia of goblet cells is observed.

It is unknown whether the anatomic site of mucosal invasion is selected haphazardly by a particular species or is influenced by a distinct organ preference. Two studies conducted 30 years apart found very similar distributions of encysted cyathostomin larvae in the intestinal tract with roughly about half the larvae in the cecum, a little over 40% present in the ventral colon, and less than 10% present in the dorsal colon (Reinemeyer and Herd, 1986; Bellaw *et al.*, 2018). A recent study conducted on 37 foals aged 50–298 days revealed a similar distribution with the exception that the proportion in the dorsal colon was higher. The proportions in that study were 44% (cecum), 37% (ventral colon), and 19% (dorsal colon) (Nielsen and Lyons, 2017). It has been reported that larvae present in the submucosa elicited a stronger inflammatory response than larvae present in the lamina propria (Steinbach *et al.*, 2006; Steuer, Loynachan, and Nielsen, submitted). Larval distribution has distinct pathologic relevance, as discussed later in this chapter.

Mucosal penetration by recently ingested L$_3$s has distinct pathologic consequences. It is logical that a macroorganism penetrating between or through mucosal epithelial cells would cause some mechanical damage. Indeed, invasion is accompanied by focal inflammation and a fibroelastic reaction in the lamina propria (Love, Murphy, and Mellor, 1999), with perhaps an immune component in sensitized horses. Experimental infections have been accompanied by changes in clinical pathology parameters as soon as three weeks post-infection, suggesting that mucosal invasion alone can be pathogenic (Love, Murphy, and Mellor, 1999). The number and cumulative severity of these lesions is expected to be greater in horses grazing heavily infective pastures, and would generally occur during seasons or climatic conditions that favor larval development and/or persistence. In addition to climatic and seasonal factors, the risk of invasive damage would be compounded by factors that increase the numbers of larvae ingested, including overstocking of pastures and limited forage height.

The negative consequences of larval invasion can be minimized by limiting the numbers of infective larvae to which grazing horses are exposed. That topic is addressed in greater detail elsewhere in this volume (Chapter 6).

Encystment

Following invasion of the mucosa, the L$_3$s of some cyathostomin species apparently penetrate no deeper than the mucosa, whereas other species invade the submucosa. In general, the latter tend to be larger cyathostomin species. Within days of mucosal penetration, a fibrous capsule of host origin develops around each invading larva, which can now be classified as "encysted" (Figure 2.5).

The cyst wall comprises the boundaries of each larva's universe for a period ranging from a few weeks to as long as 2.5 years (Gibson, 1953). Encysted larvae are constantly surrounded by a small volume of clear fluid, but the properties of this liquid are unknown. The cyst wall apparently allows two-way passage of soluble materials. Because larvae increase greatly in size and maturity during their period of residence, it is obvious that nutrients of host origin must be able to penetrate the fibrous capsule. In addition, certain excretory products of the larva must be able to pass in the opposite direction because space within the cyst is insufficient to contain the volume that must be produced over 2 or more years. Regardless, the host's protective mechanisms seem fairly oblivious to the presence of encysted larvae. Histopathology of mucosal stages reveals only modest inflammation around the cyst wall, as long as the structure remains intact (Love, Murphy, and Mellor, 1999) (Figure 2.6).

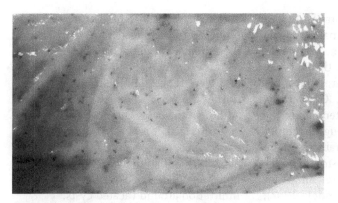

Figure 2.5 Normal gross appearance of encysted cyathostomins within the cecal mucosa of a clinically healthy horse. Each dot represents one encysted larva.

(A)   (B)

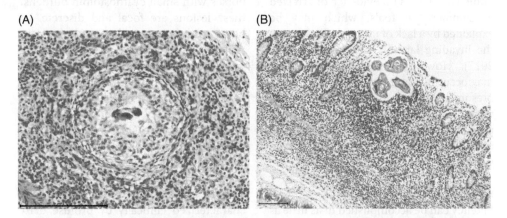

Figure 2.6 Histopathology sections of encysted cyathostomin larvae within the large intestinal walls (hematoxylin and eosin). (A) L_3 larva in the submucosa surrounded by local inflammatory cells and a thin fibrous connective tissue capsule. There is a large population of lymphocytes and macrophages present, along with a few eosinophils. (B) L_4 larva located in the mucosa. The larva is surrounded by a thin fibrous capsule and a large population of eosinophils and lymphocytes. Size bars: both 100 μm. (*Source:* Photograph courtesy of Dr. Alan Loynachan).

Another functional aspect is that the fibrous cyst capsule apparently prevents the entry of some types of anthelmintics. For example, pyrimidine salts and ivermectin have no apparent efficacy against encysted larval stages, regardless of dosage (see Chapter 7).

Some portion of the encysted larval population may reside within the gut tissues for 2 years or longer (Gibson, 1953), as a consequence of a process known as arrested development. Arrested development is defined as a temporary cessation of parasitic development, at a specific stage in the life cycle, in response to certain environmental, host, or parasite factors. Only when arrest is terminated can the parasite resume progressive development to the adult stage and, ultimately, sexual reproduction. Arrested development has been adopted by numerous nematode species and is generally considered a survival strategy to avoid conditions that disfavor the immediate propagation of a successive generation. Cyathostomins arrest at the EL_3 stage, apparently to evade harsh climatic conditions that are inimical to the development and survival of infective stages in the environment. Accordingly, small strongyle populations in a northern temperate climate are likely to arrest through the winter months, emerging as fresh juveniles in late winter and spring. Conversely, cyathostomins in southern temperate climates tend to arrest through summer months to avoid high temperatures. There is some evidence that cyathostomin populations in equatorial climates may not arrest at all (Eysker and Pandey, 1987), presumably because local conditions are perennially favorable for translation. Similarly, there is no evidence of arrested development in foals, which may be explained by a lack of immune response to the invading larvae (Nielsen and Lyons, 2017). However, arrested development may occur in mature horses at any season, presumably due to host immune responses. Arrest is not an all-or-none phenomenon; it may involve only a portion of the worm population and might even vary by species.

Excystment

Patency can be accomplished in as little as 5 to 6 weeks, as often observed in foals. However, this can only occur when cyathostomin larvae undergo progressive maturation, *i.e.*, they develop directly and without interruption from an infective L_3 to the adult stage. In an uninterrupted life cycle, the residence of larvae in the encysted stage is effectively limited to less than one month.

Emerging larvae presumably break through the cyst wall by means of a combination of mechanical and chemical factors, although none of the latter has been described. Emergence of larvae from mucosal cysts (*i.e.*, "excystment") is the single most pathogenic event of the cyathostomin life cycle. Late fourth stage larvae are 10 or more times larger than early L_3s, so considerably greater mechanical damage to the mucosa ensues than when larvae first invaded as newly ingested L_3s. A substantial host reaction is mounted to this mechanical damage, but even greater is the putative host response to the excretory and secretory materials that were sequestered within the capsule during the period of larval development. Although the cyst contents have not been characterized, it is likely that they contain cytokines or other bioactive materials that elicit host inflammation; Love, Murphy, and Mellor (1999) describe eosinophilic infiltration around vacated cysts.

Sites of recent larval excystment exhibit hemorrhage, congestion, and edema. In horses with small cyathostomin burdens, these lesions are focal and discrete. In horses with large populations, lesions are multiple and often coalescent. Horses with very large cyathostomin populations may exhibit massive inflammation of the large intestine. The mucosa can become extremely edematous, 1 to 2 cm thick, and hemorrhagic or necrotic. The clinical syndrome associated with these findings is termed larval cyathostominosis (Love, Murphy, and Mellor, 1999; Peregrine *et al.*, 2006). This syndrome is characterized clinically by profuse diarrhea, dehydration, weight loss, hypoproteinemia, and ventral edema. Laboratory diagnostics may also reveal dehydration, neutrophilia, and anemia. Ultrasonography can be employed to measure the thickness of large intestinal walls, and exaggerated mural dimensions would support the diagnosis.

Larval cyathostominosis (LC) occurs in all ages, but is more prevalent in horses between one and four years of age. LC has a distinct, seasonal distribution, which coincides with the expected patterns of larval emergence from encystment. Thus, LC is most common in late winter/early spring in northern climates (Reid *et al.*, 1995) and presumably in late summer in warmer climates. Larval cyathostominosis can be compared to winter (Type II) ostertagiosis in cattle and usually occurs in single animals within a herd.

Management and deworming practices are important contributing factors to the incidence of LC, but given the uneven distribution of parasites within a herd, some horses will always be at more risk than others. The case fatality rate is reported to be around 50% (Love, Murphy, and Mellor, 1999), but considering that all horses have cyathostomin infections, LC remains a rare event.

A less acute clinical presentation is also attributed to excysting cyathostomin larvae. In these cases, horses typically exhibit variable fecal consistency over an extended period of time. This can be accompanied by weight loss and subnormal to low plasma protein concentrations, but these findings are much less pronounced than observed in classic LC.

In some cases of LC, newly emerged cyathostomin larvae are present in the feces, often in large numbers, but this occurs in healthy horses as well. Thus, no single clinical sign is pathognomonic and a definitive diagnosis can be difficult to reach (see Chapter 9).

A marked, seasonal distribution notwithstanding, the single most important risk factor for LC is anthelmintic treatment within one to two weeks prior to the onset of disease (Reid *et al.*, 1995). The rapid kill and removal of luminal parasites appears to trigger a synchronous emergence of encysted larval stages from the mucosal lining, presumably as a function of population dynamics to replace the recently removed adults. The majority of excystment lesions are observed in the cecum and ventral colon, which is consistent with the known distribution of cyathostomin encystment. In typical infections, the mucosa of the dorsal colon (DC) remains relatively unaffected and pathologists may consider it as an internal reference standard for a "normal, unaffected" gut. Numerous adult and late fourth stage larval cyathostomins preferentially inhabit the lumen of the DC, but their presence does not appear to change the gross appearance or inflammatory status of the DC mucosa.

Although signs of mucosal inflammation have been observed following anthelmintic treatment (Reinemeyer, 2003; Steinbach *et al.*, 2006), the general consensus is that these reactions are subtle, if they can be measured at all (Nielsen *et al.*, 2015; Steuer, Loynachan, and Nielsen, submitted). Evaluations of systemic concentrations of acute phase markers and pro-inflammatory cytokine gene expression have found very few fluctuations that can be associated with either experimental inoculation with strongyle parasites (Andersen *et al.*, 2014) or anthelmintic treatment of naturally acquired cyathostomin infections (Nielsen *et al.*, 2013). Recent research has documented that intestinal nematodes are capable of reducing the inflammatory response by modulating host immunity (McKay, 2009). This factor may explain the limited inflammatory reactions associated with cyathostomin infection in clinically healthy horses.

Adults

Adult cyathostomins are considered to be relatively innocuous, even when present in extremely high numbers. Although some species may attach weakly to the mucosa, most reside in the paramucosal ingesta, where they feed on particulate organic materials. The gut contents of mature cyathostomins have been shown to contain ciliate protozoa and even strongyle eggs.

Many cyathostomin species are known to exhibit distinct site/organ preferences as adults. For example, *Cylicostephanus longibursatus* adults occupy the dorsal colon (DC) almost exclusively, and often in very large numbers, whereas *Petrovinema poculatum* is rarely observed outside the cecum (see Table 1.1). Interestingly, the dorsal colon can be heavily populated by adult cyathostomins, as one study found the DC to harbor 50%

of the luminal cyathostomin burden, which was substantially more than the cecum (7%) or ventral colon (42%) (Bellaw *et al.*, 2018). The same study found the encysted larval burden to be differently distributed, with 49%, 43%, and 8% recovered from the cecum, ventral colon, and dorsal colon, respectively. This strongly suggests that site/organ preferences are effected only after excystment and emergence of the late L_4s.

Chronic cyathostominosis has been described, and it is a different clinical syndrome than larval cyathostominosis. Whereas the latter is specifically associated with mass emergence of mucosal larvae, chronic cyathostominosis is generally related to the cumulative effects of the multiple parasitic stages which occupy a host contemporaneously (Love, Murphy, and Mellor, 1999). Symptoms are nonspecific, but include weight loss, dull haircoat, pot-bellied appearance, colic, and loose feces. Hypoproteinemia may be present, but is not a consistent finding.

Parascaris spp.

Because the life cycle of *Parascaris* involves migration within the host, this nematode has the potential to damage more than one organ system. After ingestion of larvated eggs, third stage larvae emerge in the lumen of the small intestine. They then migrate through the wall of the small intestine, enter local lymphatics, and are carried to the liver. Larvae migrate within the liver for approximately one week, resulting in inflammatory tracts and white, fibrous scars under the liver capsule, reminiscent of those caused by *Ascaris suum* in swine. Third stage larvae leave the liver approximately one week after infection and are carried to the pulmonary circulation via the posterior vena cava. Larvae are trapped in terminal pulmonary arterioles or capillaries, rupture the vessel wall and enter alveoli, causing focal eosinophilic inflammation with edema and hemorrhage. Larvae migrate

proximally within the airways or are coughed up into the pharynx. Migrating larvae have generally left the lungs by 2 to 3 weeks post-infection. Ascarid larvae are swallowed and return to the gut, where they develop progressively from fourth stage larvae to adults within the small intestine. Adult ascarids may survive for several months and continue to increase in size after achieving sexual maturity.

Migration of larval ascarids through pulmonary tissues (2 to 4 weeks after infection) may be accompanied by frequent coughing, and a grayish-white, purulent nasal discharge (Srihakim and Swerczek, 1978; Clayton and Duncan, 1978). The presence of ascarids in the alimentary tract may be accompanied by decreased feed intake, diarrhea, poor growth, rough hair coat, and weight loss or poor weight gain. Ascarids do not attach to the mucosa, but apparently compete with the host for digested nutrients. Historical work with radioisotopes demonstrated that parasitized foals had greater total body water and lower total body solids than control animals (Clayton, Duncan, and Dargie, 1980). Infected foals also had lower serum concentrations and body pools of albumin.

Ascarids occasionally cause small intestinal obstructions, especially as a consequence of recent anthelmintic treatment. A review of 52 published cases of ascarid small intestinal impaction revealed an equal distribution of males and females with a median age of five months, but the condition did occur in horses as old as two years. Of the 37 cases that underwent surgery, 31 survived to discharge, but only 11 survived beyond one year after the incident (Nielsen, 2016a). Intestinal rupture was found in seven cases and other complications included intussusception (4) and volvulus (8). Effective anthelmintic treatment of a foal with a large ascarid burden appears to constitute a risk factor for impaction, as discussed further in Chapter 7.

Practitioners should always be concerned about the possibility of ascarid impaction whenever history, clinical signs, or diagnostic results suggest that an individual juvenile might be harboring a large ascarid burden (see Chapter 7). No adverse events have been reported as a result of killing ascarid larvae as they migrate through the liver and lungs.

Oxyuris equi

Following ingestion of larvated eggs, third stage larval (L$_3$) *Oxyuris* invade the mucosal crypts of the cecum and ventral colon, where they develop to the L$_4$ stage. Fourth stage larvae then emerge and feed on the mucosa until they mature into adults. Local mucosal inflammation has been reported to accompany larval invasion, but the clinical consequences of these observations appear to be minimal. Indeed, it would be difficult to discriminate such lesions from the more prevalent and numerous cyathostomin-induced lesions in the same tissues.

Adult pinworms are generally found in the dorsal colon. They do not attach to the mucosa and their only routine pathology is secondary irritation from oviposition. Females migrate through the descending colon and rectum to discharge eggs on to the perianal skin of the host in a proteinaceous fluid. It is believed that the females die shortly after this event, and pinworms are only rarely recovered from the rectum (Reinemeyer and Nielsen, 2014). As the proteinaceous fluid dries, it apparently becomes irritating to the host. Consequently, horses rub their tail heads and rumps against fixed objects, causing local damage to the skin, haircoat, and tail. Horses rub their tails for numerous other reasons, so this behavior is not pathognomonic for pinworm infection.

Tapeworms

When present in large numbers, *Anoplocephala perfoliata* can cause severe inflammation at attachment sites around the ileocecal junction (Figure 2.7). Ulceration of the mucosa with formation of pseudomembranes has been reported, along with fibrosis of the muscularis layers of the cecum, and even transmural inflammation of the adventitial layer. Abattoir surveys have related tapeworm burdens to the degree of local pathological damage (Kjær *et al.*, 2007; Williamson *et al.*, 1997), but there is no corresponding evidence that correlates the degree of mucosal damage to clinical signs. Tapeworm burdens of 20 adult *A. perfoliata* or fewer generally cause little mucosal damage. Additional theories have been advanced that equine tapeworms

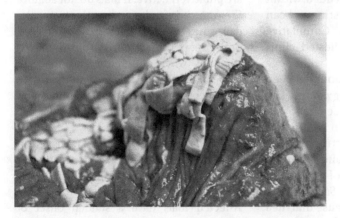

Figure 2.7 Adult *Anoplocephala perfoliata* attached to the intestinal wall at their predilection site around the ileocecal valve.

hinder alimentary motility (peristalsis) by interfering with the local autonomic nervous supply of the gut (Pavone *et al.*, 2011).

Numerous case reports have associated tapeworm infection with ileocecal intussusception and even intestinal rupture (Barclay, Phillips, and Foerner, 1982; Owen, Jagger, and Quan-Taylor, 1989). Several case-control studies have clearly documented the role of *A. perfoliata* as a risk factor for colic associated with the ileal region (Nielsen, 2016b). These ileal conditions include impactions and intussusceptions. One study also found an association with spasmodic colic (Proudman, French, and Trees, 1998), but this has yet to be corroborated. Several investigations in which broader definitions of colic were used did not identify any associations with *A. perfoliata* (Nielsen, 2016b). Although intestinal parasites can be associated with specific and strictly defined colic types, the colic complex is indeed multifactorial and difficult to associate with a specific pathogen.

Strongyloides

Strongyloides westeri infections can be established during the first weeks of life when foals ingest infective larvae while suckling, and patent infections have been reported in foals as young as five days old (Dewes, 1989).

Parasitic females are embedded within the mucosa of the small intestine and can cause local inflammation. Cumulative gut irritation may be manifested clinically as diarrhea, especially with large worm burdens. A correlation between diarrhea and high *Strongyloides* egg counts (>2000 EPG) has been reported (Netherwood *et al.*, 1996). In addition to diarrhea, foals with clinical strongyloidosis can display anorexia and lethargy. Experimental inoculation of foals with very high doses of infective *Strongyloides* larvae has been shown to cause diarrhea and in some cases death (Lyons, Drudge, and Tolliver, 1973).

A common differential for a diagnosis of strongyloidosis is foal heat diarrhea (FHD), which typically begins during the second week of life. Apart from loose stools and "scalding" of the skin on the hindquarters, however, foals with FHD are otherwise normal. They suckle well and remain alert and active. Because most *Strongyloides* infections remain asymptomatic, the observation of *S. westeri* eggs in a fecal sample from a young foal with diarrhea is by no means a clear-cut demonstration of cause and effect.

Specific anthelmintic treatment should be reserved for symptomatic cases of *Strongyloides* infection. Routine deworming of foals at 1 to 2 weeks of age to prevent or mitigate *Strongyloides* infections is unnecessary from a health standpoint and therefore discouraged. Similarly, little benefit is gained by treating the mare with a macrocyclic lactone in the last month of gestation, with the intention of preventing lactogenic transmission to the foal. Mares apparently harbor dormant *Strongyloides* larvae within the abdominal wall and it is unknown when they resume activity and begin to migrate to the mammary gland. Anthelmintic treatments are unlikely to be very effective against dormant larvae, so some veterinarians and farm managers choose to treat the mares right at foaling, when *Strongyloides* larvae are putatively active. If foals do not acquire *S. westeri* infections directly from the dam, they are still likely to be infected orally or percutaneously from the environment when the mare and foal are turned out to pasture. *Strongyloides* infections occur sporadically in weanlings and yearlings as well, but at considerably lower infection intensities.

A so-called "frenzy" syndrome has been described in foals and is associated with massive percutaneous penetration by *Strongyloides* L_3 stages (Dewes, 1989). Affected foals have a sudden onset of stamping, walking quickly, circling and rolling in the mud, and scratching the face, ears, and neck with their hind feet. Episodes were 35 minutes or less in duration. Similar symptoms of distress were also noted in mares.

Foals appear to develop acquired immunity between the time of weaning and about 8–10 months of age. However, strongyloidosis should not be considered as a differential for clinical diarrhea in weanlings or older juveniles.

The prevalence of *S. westeri* infections has reportedly changed over the past decades. Three surveys conducted between 1992 and 2004 reported that *Strongyloides* eggs were found in the feces of only 1.5–6% of foals examined (Lyons *et al.*, 1993; Lyons and Tolliver, 2004; Lyons, Tolliver, and Collins, 2006). This was considered a dramatic reduction from historical prevalences of ~90% and was largely attributed to the widespread use of effective anthelmintics (Lyons and Tolliver, 2014a). Recent investigations, however, have suggested a resurgence in the prevalence of patent infections in suckling foals, suggesting that anthelmintic treatments may not be as effective as previously believed. Lyons and Tolliver (2014b) reported positive fecal results in 15% of foals born in central Kentucky during 2013. A follow-up study conducted during 2014 reported that fecal examinations were positive in 28% of colts and 33% of fillies aged 17–117 days (Lyons and Tolliver, 2014a). One of these studies did not find any apparent differences in foals out of mares that were dewormed close to foaling compared to foals out of mares that were not (Lyons and Tolliver, 2014a). A plausible explanation for this resurgence of *S. westeri* in foals could be the diminished use of ivermectin in this age group fostered by concerns about widespread resistance to this drug in *Parascaris* spp. (see Chapter 8) (Lyons and Tolliver, 2014b).

Lungworms

Lungworm infection in horses is characterized by a chronic, productive cough, mucopurulent nasal discharge, and occasional fever. Clinical cases invariably feature a history of sharing pasture with one or more donkeys. The most pronounced pathologic finding is eosinophilic bronchitis, which, if chronic and severe, can result in a significant loss of lung function. As opposed to donkeys, horses are unsuitable definitive hosts for *Dictyocaulus arnfieldi*, so no or very few reproductive stages are produced to assist in diagnosis (see Chapter 9). However, some populations of working horses are reported to pass eggs or larvae in the feces (Maria, Shahardar, and Bushra, 2012), perhaps because of their frequent, close association with donkeys and mules. Eosinophilia may be detected by transtracheal wash or alveolar lavage, but is not pathognomonic for lungworm infection. Infected horses generally respond well to therapy with macrocyclic lactone anthelmintics. A comprehensive management program would require treatment of resident donkeys and segregation of horse and donkey pastures in the future.

Trichostrongylus axei

Larval *T. axei* develop within gastric glands and adults live in close contact with the mucosa of the glandular portion of the equine stomach. As in ruminants, the presence of large numbers of *T. axei* results in proliferation and hypertrophy of the gastric mucosa. Trichostrongylosis is not known to affect gastric pH in horses and levels of plasma pepsinogen were not increased in infected horses in one study (Herd, 1986). Although populations of *Trichostrongylus* can be maintained and perpetuated by horse herds, severe infections usually occur only in horses with a history of co-grazing pastures with cattle or other ruminants.

Stomach worms (*Habronema* and *Draschia*)

Habronema spp. live in intimate contact with the gastric mucosa, but the adult stages are not known to cause clinical signs. In contrast, *Draschia* adults cause the formation of large, tumor-like nodules at the *margo plicatus*, but this parasite has virtually disappeared from North American horses in the past two decades. Otherwise, gastric infections have few manifestations. Cutaneous habronemiasis/draschiasis occurs when larvae enter skin wounds or mucocutaneous junctions to cause persistent, granulomatous lesions known as summer sores. Biopsies of suspected habronemiasis lesions reveal eosinophilia, fibrous connective tissue, secondary bacterial infection, and ulceration. Cutaneous lesions can be treated with systemic macrocyclic lactone anthelmintics or excised surgically, but numerous alternative approaches have been employed in the past (Sellon, 2007).

A pulmonary form of habronemiasis has been described (Schuster *et al.*, 2010). A horse was euthanatized due to acute respiratory problems and the lung exhibited multiple abscesses containing *Habronema* spp. larvae. It is unknown how the larvae arrived in the lungs and whether this pulmonary form is an underdiagnosed condition in horses.

Eyeworms

Thelazia lacrymalis is reported to infect conjunctival *cul de sacs* of horses on pasture (Lyons, Tolliver, and Collins, 2006). Although infections are generally asymptomatic, cases of mild conjunctivitis and keratitis have been reported. One study reported abscess-forming dacryoadenitis in a stallion with chronic, recurrent bilateral conjunctivitis (Wollanke, Gerhards, and Pfleghaar, 2004). Other infectious and allergic etiologies can cause similar clinical signs, so multiple differential diagnoses exist.

Onchocerca

As adults, the three species of *Onchocerca* occurring in horses reside in the nuchal ligament or connective tissues of the distal limbs. The location in the nuchal liga-

ment has given rise to the common name "neck threadworm". Fibrous nodules occasionally form around the resident parasites in either location and dystrophic calcification has been observed. However, the presence of adult parasites has not been associated with adverse clinical consequences.

Onchocerca spp. reproduce by forming microfilariae that congregate in the skin, where they are ingested by arthropod intermediate hosts of the genera *Culicoides* (midges) or *Simulium* (black flies). Microfilariae rarely may cause eye lesions. The most common clinical manifestation is chronic dermatitis, which may be confused with allergic dermatitis (*i.e.*, summer eczema) caused by hypersensitivity to *Culicoides* bites. Lesions of cutaneous onchocerciasis may persist perennially or may increase in severity during seasons when the arthropod vectors are actively feeding. The typical location for lesions associated with microfilariae is along the ventral midline of the horse. Systemic treatment with macrocyclic lactones is reported to have good efficacy against microfilariae, but up to 25% of treated horses experience pruritus or ventral edema in response to dead or dying microfilariae. Although not technically adulticidal, treatment with macrocyclic lactones apparently renders adult worms infertile for several months. Production of microfilariae inevitably resumes at some interval after M/L therapy, so repeated treatments may be necessary for long-term management of skin disease (Sellon, 2007).

Setaria

Setaria are large, filarioid nematodes that are usually found free within the peritoneal cavity. These relatively large worms cause no apparent damage, although elevated levels of eosinophils can be found by abdominocentesis and in blood samples. However, the latter may be associated with the microfilarial stage, which is present in the blood stream. Generally, *Setaria* adults have no pathologic significance unless they wander into aberrant sites, such as the eye or central nervous system.

Arthropods

Gasterophilus spp.

First instar bots occupy fissures on the surface of the tongue and second instar bots reside in gingival pockets at the base of molar teeth. These stages have recently been associated with primary parasitic periodontitis, characterized by lingual lesions, necrosis of gingival papillae, and deepened periodontal pockets. Affected horses exhibit clinical signs such as excessive salivation, lingual irritation, and chewing problems (Osterman Lind, Chirico, and Lundstrom, 2012). Second and third instars of *G. intestinalis* are typically found attached to the mucosa of the non-glandular stomach (Figure 2.8), while those of *G. nasalis* are affixed to the mucosa of the duodenal ampulla, just distal to the pylorus. Attachment sites are characterized by large (1–2 mm) pits surrounded by hypertrophic mucosa. Lesions at attachment sites apparently have little negative impact on the host. Investigations

report that the depth of penetration in the gastric or duodenal walls is minimal and that proliferation of tissues beneath the ulcers counteracts thinning of the walls, making perforation highly unlikely (Cogley and Cogley, 1999). The greatest negative impact of bot flies on their hosts might be the agitation horses experience during oviposition by females.

General impact of parasitism

Loss or diversion of nutrients

At the beginning of this chapter, we presented a partial list of abnormal clinical signs often attributed to parasitism. To that collection, we might add negative impacts on productivity and performance parameters, which vary widely for different types of horses. Performance for athletes differs from that of brood stock, and halter and conformation classes have different and unique requirements. In any case, these many and varied effects all require careful measurement and comparison; subjective assessments are not sufficient "proof" of parasitic damage. Many of the purported negative effects of parasitism on productivity are similar, if not identical, to those caused by nutritional

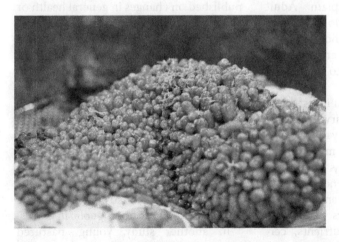

Figure 2.8 *Gasterophilus intestinalis* larvae attached to the non-glandular portion of the gastric mucosa.

problems. Therefore, it is possible that parasitism exerts many of its general effects by interfering with the digestion, distribution, or utilization of nutrients, or that it limits the use of nutrients to maintaining homeostasis rather than contributing to anabolic outcomes, such as increased bone and muscle mass, athletic fitness, etc.

This seems a logical hypothesis, but the only equine parasite for which interference with host utilization of nutrients has been documented is *Parascaris*. These very large worms physically compete with the host for the use of digested nutrients (amino acids, simple carbohydrates, and lipids) within the small intestine. Ascarids have been shown to ingest radiolabeled methionine when administered orally to infected foals (Clayton, Duncan, and Dargie, 1980). The impact of ascarid infection may be more dramatic because its prevalence coincides precisely with a rapid growth phase of the horse's lifespan. Foals harboring large numbers of roundworms simply cannot access the nutritional building blocks for optimal growth, metabolism, or performance.

Although nutritional deprivation or redirection are tempting hypotheses for other helminth infections of mature horses (cyathostomins, primarily), this is largely unsupported by facts and therefore much harder to explain. Adult cyathostomins apparently do not derive nutrients directly from the host mucosa, unlike large strongyles, and are relatively non-pathogenic compared to their larval stages within host tissues.

An issue that has not been investigated is the impact of encysted larvae on host nutrient cycling. Encysted cyathostomins increase in size 10-fold or more during their development from EL_3s to late L_4s, and the duration of residence of these resource burners may extend through many months, if not years. Nematode growth requires critical nutrients, certainly amino acids and energy sources, and those are obviously derived from elements ingested by the host. Virtually nothing is known of the processes by which the cyst wall permits the influx of nutrients and the excretion of waste products. Regardless of the mechanisms, most adult horses harbor literally thousands of encysted larvae, all of which utilize host nutrients on a constant basis. This implies that fewer critical nutrients would be available to support homeostatic and anabolic processes of the host.

Another potential source of nutrient loss is associated with excystment of late fourth stage larvae. The mucosal disruptions caused by excysting larvae initially hemorrhage, and presumably leak plasma thereafter until healed. This is a focal form of protein-losing enteropathy, and the host probably cannot recover plasma proteins spilling into the lumen of the large intestine. No digestive enzymes operate in the posterior gut to degrade insoluble proteins into simple amino acids that could feasibly cross the mucosa. Regardless of whether host protein is passed in the feces or degraded by local gut flora, it is no longer available to the horse.

Clinical health and productivity

Surprisingly little information has been published on changes in general health or production parameters in response to anthelmintic treatment or other effective forms of parasite control. One long-term study investigated the incidence of colic in populations of horses kept under different anthelmintic treatment regimens, and concluded that the use of macrocyclic lactones was associated with a lower incidence of colic (Uhlinger, 1990). Coprocultures indicated an absence of large strongyles in these horses, so this suggests that small strongyle infection constitutes a risk factor for colic in horses.

In another study, young, pastured horses that were treated with moxidectin or ivermectin achieved greater weight gains than an untreated control group (Reinemeyer and Clymer, 2002), although the observed differences were not significant ($P < 0.05$) until 120 days post-treatment. A number of studies have evaluated body condition scores of horses and reported a positive association with anthelmintic treatment (Matthee *et al.*, 2002; Crane *et al.*, 2010; Reinemeyer *et al.*, 2014). One recent study followed three populations of Thoroughbred foals from birth until they were taken to the sales as 16 month old yearlings. Despite clear evidence of anthelmintic resistance and obvious differences between the two anthelmintic regimens evaluated, growth rates and body condition scores were found to be at or above industry standards (Bellaw *et al.*, 2016). This serves to illustrate that suboptimal parasite control can be compensated by good management and well-balanced diets. Clinicians often report that cases of parasitic disease or ill-thrift are more likely to occur in situations where management is less than optimal. High stocking density, low quality food resources, and the presence of other diseases are often observed to be predisposing factors. This is in agreement with studies with working equids that spend a significant proportion of the day doing physical work and often have access to very poor nutrition (Yoseph *et al.*, 2005).

Traditional notions that horses gain weight or improve body condition rapidly after effective deworming are unwarranted and simply inaccurate. (The converse reveals the fallacy behind subjective assessments that an anthelmintic treatment had obviously failed because the horse did not "slick up" or gain weight soon after treatment.)

One study investigated strongyle fecal egg counts of Standardbred Trotters and evaluated the potential association with race performance. Surprisingly, the more successful racers had a significant tendency toward higher egg counts (Fog, Vigre, and Nielsen, 2011). In other words, the horses in this study appeared to be unaffected by the presence of moderate strongyle burdens. The effects of parasitism on other types of performance have not been documented objectively in horses, nor have improvements thereof in response to anthelmintic treatment or other control measures been described in any detail. Yet, persistent presumptions to the contrary support many traditional practices, including frequent deworming of race horses, use of daily, preventive dewormers in halter horses, etc. Objectively, there is very little proof one way or the other. These are classic examples of uncontrolled experiments: "I always do thus and so, and I'm happy with the (putative) results, so it obviously works." Therein lies perhaps the greatest obstacle to changing prevalent attitudes about the importance and methods of parasite control.

References

Andersen, U.V., Reinemeyer, C.R., Toft, N., *et al.* (2014) Physiologic and systemic acute phase inflammatory responses in young horses repeatedly infected with cyathostomins and *Strongylus vulgaris*. *Vet. Parasitol.*, 201, 67–74.

Barclay, W., Phillips, T., and Foerner, J. (1982) Intussusception associated with *Anoplocephala perfoliata* infection in five horses. *J. Am. Vet. Med. Assoc.*, 180, 752–753.

Bellaw, J.L., Pagan, J., Cadell, S., *et al.* (2016) Objective evaluation of two deworming regimens in young Thoroughbreds using parasitological and performance parameters. *Vet. Parasitol.*, 221, 69–75.

Bellaw J.L., Krebs, K., Reinemeyer, C.R., *et al.* (2018) Anthelmintic therapy of equine cyathostomin nematodes – larvicidal efficacy, egg reappearance period, and drug resistance. *Int. J. Parasitol.*, 48, 97–105.

Clayton, H.M. and Duncan, J.L. (1978) Clinical signs associated with *Parascaris equorum* infection in worm-free pony foals and yearlings. *Vet. Parasitol.*, 4, 69.

Clayton, H.M., Duncan, J.L., and Dargie, J.D. (1980) Pathophysiological changes associated with *Parascaris equorum* infection in the foal. *Equine Vet. J.*, 12, 23–25.

Cogley, T.P. and Cogley, M.C. (1999) Inter-relationship between *Gasterophilus* larvae and the horse's gastric and duodenal wall with special reference to penetration. *Vet. Parasitol.*, 86, 127–142.

Crane, M.A., Khallaayoune, K., Scantlebury, C., and Christley, R.M. (2010) A randomized triple blind trial to assess the effect of an anthelmintic programme for working equids in Morocco. *BMC Vet. Res.*, 7, 1.

Davies, G., Stear, M.J., Benothman, M., et al. (2006) Quantitative trait loci associated with parasitic infection in Scottish blackface sheep. *Heredity*, 96, 252–258.

Dewes, H.F. (1989) The association between weather, frenzied behavior, percutaneous invasion by *Strongyloides westeri* larvae and *Rhodococcus equi* disease in foals. *N. Z. Vet. J.*, 37, 69.

Drudge, J.H. (1972) Endoparasitisms, in *Equine Medicine and Surgery*, 2nd edn, American Veterinary Publications Inc., Illinois, USA, pp. 157–179.

Duncan, J.L. and Pirie, H.M. (1975) The pathogenesis of single experimental infections with *Strongylus vulgaris* in foals. *Res. Vet. Sci.*, 18, 82–93.

Enigk, K. (1951) Die Pathogenese der thrombotisch-embolischen Kolik des Pferdes. *Monatsh. Prakt. Tierheilk.*, 3, 65–74.

Eysker, M. and Pandey, V.S. (1987) Overwintering of nonmigrating strongyles in donkeys in the highveld of Zimbabwe. *Res. Vet. Sci.*, 42, 262–263.

Fog, P., Vigre, H., and Nielsen, M.K. (2011) Strongyle egg counts in Standardbred trotters: Are they associated with race performance? *Equine Vet. J.*, 43, 89–92.

Gasbarre, L.C., Leighton, E.A., and Davies, C.J. (1990) Genetic control of immunity to gastrointestinal nematodes of cattle. *Vet. Parasitol.* 37, 257–272.

Gibson, T.E. (1953) The effect of repeated anthelmintic treatment with phenothiazine on fecal egg counts of housed horses, with some observations on the life cycle of *Trichonema* spp. in the horse. *J. Helminthol.*, 27, 29–40.

Herd, R.P. (1986) Serum pepsinogen concentrations of ponies naturally infected with *Trichostrongylus axei*. *Equine Vet. J.*, 18 (6), 490–491.

Jaskoski, B.J. and Colglazier, M.L. (1956) A report of *Strongylus asini* from the United States. *J. Am. Vet. Med. Assoc.*, 129, 513–514.

Kjær, L.N., Lungholt, M.M., Nielsen, M.K., *et al.* (2007) Interpretation of serum antibody response to *Anoplocephala perfoliata* in relation to parasite burden and faecal egg count. *Equine Vet. J.*, 39, 529–533.

Love, S., Murphy, D., and Mellor, D. (1999) Pathogenicity of cyathostome infection. *Vet. Parasitol.*, 85, 113–122.

Lyons, E.T. and Tolliver, S.C. (2004) Prevalence of parasite eggs (*Strongyloides westeri, Parascaris equorum*, and strongyles) and oocysts (*Eimeria leuckarti*) in the feces of Thoroughbred foals on 14 farms in central Kentucky in 2003. *Parasitol. Res.*, 92, 400–404.

Lyons, E.T. and Tolliver, S.C. (2014a) Prevalence of patent *Strongyloides westeri* infections in Thoroughbred foals in 2014. *Parasitol. Res.*, 113, 4163–4164.

Lyons, E.T. and Tolliver, S.C. (2014b) *Strongyloides westeri* and *Parascaris equorum*: Observations in field studies in Thoroughbred foals on some farms in Central Kentucky, USA. *Helminthologia*, 51, 7–12.

Lyons, E.T., Drudge, J.H., and Tolliver, S.C. (1973) Life-cycle of *Strongyloides westeri* in equine. *J. Parasitol.*, 59, 780–787.

Lyons, E.T., Tolliver, S.C., and Collins, S.S. (2006) Prevalence of large endoparasites at necropsy in horses infected with Population B small strongyles in a herd established in Kentucky in 1966. *Parasitol. Res.*, 99, 114–118.

Lyons, E.T., Tolliver, S.C., Drudge, J.H., *et al.* (1993) Natural infections of *Strongyloides westeri*: prevalence in horse foals on several farms in central Kentucky in 1992. *Vet. Parasitol.*, 50, 101–107.

Maria, A., Shahardar, R.A., and Bushra, M. (2012) Prevalence of gastrointestinal helminth parasites of equines in central zone of Kashmir Valley. *Indian J. Anim. Sci.*, 82, 1276–1280.

Matthee, S., Krecek, R.C., Milne, S.A., *et al.* (2002) Impact of management interventions on helminth levels, and body and blood measurements in working donkeys in South Africa. *Vet. Parasitol.*, 107, 103–113.

McCraw, B.M. and Slocombe, J.O.D. (1978) *Strongylus edentatus*: Development and lesions from ten weeks postinfection to patency. *Can. J. Comp. Med.*, 42, 340–356.

McCraw, B.M. and Slocombe, J.O.D. (1984) *Strongylus equinus*: Development and pathological effects in the equine host. *Can. J. Comp. Med.*, 49, 372–383.

McKay, D.M. (2009) The therapeutic helminth? *Trends Parasitol.*, 25, 109–114.

Netherwood, T., Wood, J.L.N., Townsend, H.G.G., *et al.* (1996) Foal diarrhoea between 1991 and 1994 in the United Kingdom associated with *Clostridium perfringens*, rotavirus, *Strongyloides westeri* and *Cryptosporidium* spp. *Epidemiol. Infect.*, 117, 375–383.

Nielsen, M.K. (2016a) Evidence-based considerations for control of *Parascaris* spp. infections in horses. *Equine Vet. Educ.*, 28, 224–231.

Nielsen, M.K. (2016b) Equine tapeworm infections – disease, diagnosis, and control. *Equine Vet. Educ.*, 28, 388–395.

Nielsen, M.K. and Lyons, E.T. (2017) Encysted cyathostomin larvae in foals – progression of stages and the effect of seasonality. *Vet. Parasitol.*, 236, 108–112.

Nielsen, M.K., Betancourt, A., Lyons, E.T., *et al.* (2013) Characterization of the inflammatory response to anthelmintic treatment in ponies naturally infected with cyathostomin parasites. *Vet. J.*, 198, 457–462.

Nielsen, M.K., Loynachan, A.T., Jacobsen, S., *et al.* (2015) Local and systemic inflammatory and immunologic reactions to cyathostomin larvicidal therapy in horses. *Vet. Imm. Immunopathol.*, 168, 203–210.

Nielsen, M.K., Jacobsen, S., Olsen, S.N., *et al.* (2016) Non-strangulating intestinal infarction associated with *Strongylus vulgaris* in referred Danish equine patients. *Equine Vet. J.*, 48, 376–379.

Ogbourne, C.P. and Duncan, J.L. (1985) *Strongylus vulgaris* in the horse: its biology and veterinary importance. *Commonwealth Institute of Parasitology*, Commonwealth Agricultural Bureaux, London, UK.

Osterman Lind, E.O., Chirico, J., and Lundstrom, T. (2012) *Gasterophilus* larvae in association with primary parasitic periodontitis. *J. Equine Vet. Sci.*, 32, S51.

Owen, R.R., Jagger, D.W., and Quan-Taylor, R. (1989) Caecal intussusceptions in horses and the significance of *Anoplocephala perfoliata*. *Vet. Rec.*, 124, 34–37.

Pavone, S., Veronesi, F., Genchi, C., *et al.* (2011) Pathological changes caused by *Anoplocephala perfoliata* in the mucosa/submucosa and in the enteric nervous system of equine ileocecal junction. *Vet. Parasitol.*, 176, 43–52.

Peregrine, A.S., McEwen, B., Bienzle, D., *et al.* (2006) Larval cyathostominosis in horses in Ontario: an emerging disease? *Can. Vet. J.*, 47, 80–82.

Pihl, T.H., Nielsen, M.K., and Jacobsen, S. (2017) Changes in hemostasis in foals naturally infected with *Strongylus vulgaris. J. Equine Vet. Sci.*, 4, 1–7.

Pihl, T.H., Nielsen, M.K., Olsen, S.N., *et al.* (in press) Non-strangulating intestinal infarctions associated with *Strongylus vulgaris*: 30 horses (2008–2016). *Equine Vet. J.*

Proudman, C.J., French, N.P., and Trees, A.J. (1998) Tapeworm infection is a significant risk factor for spasmodic colic and ileal impaction colic in the horse. *Equine Vet. J.*, 30, 194–199.

Reid, S.W., Mair, T.S., Hillyer, M.H., and Love, S. (1995) Epidemiological risk factors associated with a diagnosis of clinical cyathostomiasis in the horse. *Equine Vet. J.*, 27, 127–130.

Reinemeyer, C.R. (2003) Indications and benefits of moxidectin use in horses. *Proceedings, World Equine Veterinary Association*, Buenos Aires, Argentina, 16 October, 2003.

Reinemeyer, C.R. and Clymer, B.C. (2002) Comparative efficiency of moxidectin gel or ivermectin paste for cyathostome control in young horses. *J. Equine Vet. Sci.*, 22, 33–36.

Reinemeyer, C.R. and Herd, R.P. (1986) Anatomic distribution of encysted cyathostome larvae in the horse. *Am. J. Vet. Res.*, 47, 510–513.

Reinemeyer, C.R. and Nielsen, M.K. (2014) Review of the biology and control of *Oxyuris equi. Equine Vet. Educ.*, 26, 584–591.

Reinemeyer, C.R., Prado, J.C., Andersen, U.V., *et al.* (2014) Effects of daily pyrantel tartrate on strongylid population dynamics and performance parameters of young horses repeatedly infected with cyathostomins and *Strongylus vulgaris. Vet. Parasitol.*, 204, 229–237.

Schuster, R.K., Sivakumar, S., Kinne, J., *et al.* (2010) Cutaneous and pulmonal habronemosis transmitted by *Musca domestica* in a stable in the United Arab Emirates. *Vet. Parasitol.*, 174, 170–174.

Sellon, D.C. (2007) Nonenteric nematodes, in *Equine Infectious Diseases* (eds D.C. Sellon and M.T. Long), Saunders Elsevier, St. Louis, MO, pp. 490–495.

Srihakim, S. and Swerczek, T.W. (1978) Pathologic changes and pathogenesis of *Parascaris equorum* infection in parasite-free pony foals. *Am. J. Vet. Res.*, 39, 1155.

Steinbach, T., Bauer, C., Sasse, H., *et al.* (2006) Small strongyle infection: Consequences of larvicidal treatment of horses with fenbendazole and moxidectin. *Vet. Parasitol.*, 139, 115–131.

Steuer, A., Loynachan, A.T., and Nielsen, M.K. (submitted) Evaluation of the mucosal inflammatory responses to larvicidal treatment.

Uhlinger, C. (1990) Effects of three anthelmintic schedules on the incidence of colic in horses. *Equine Vet. J.*, 22, 251–254.

White, N.A. (1985) Thromboembolism colic in horses. *Comp. Cont. Educ. Pract. Vet.*, 7, S156.

Williamson, R.M.C., Gasser, R.B., Middleton, D., and Beveridge, I. (1997) The distribution of *Anoplocephala perfoliata* in the intestine of the horse and associated pathological changes. *Vet. Parasitol.*, 73, 225–241.

Wollanke, B., Gerhards, H., and Pfleghaar, S. (2004) Chronic recurrent conjunctivitis due to *Thelazia lacrymalis*-induced, chronic abscess forming dacryoadenitis in a Warmblood stallion. *Pferdeheilk.*, 20, 131–134.

Wright, A.I. (1972) Verminous arteritis as a cause of colic in the horse. *Equine Vet. J.* 4, 169–174.

Yoseph, S., Smith, D.G., Mengistu, A., *et al.* (2005) Seasonal variation in the parasite burden and body condition of working donkeys in East Shewa and West Shewa regions of Ethiopia. *Trop. Anim. Health Prod.*, 37, 35–45.

3

Environmental Factors Affecting Parasite Transmission

Contributing authors: Dave Leathwick and Christian Sauermann

As mentioned in Chapter 1, a key feature of parasite propagation is that offspring must visit the environment to undergo essential changes before they are capable of infecting a new generation of hosts. Thus, the ability of eggs passed in the feces to hatch and develop to an infective stage is strongly influenced by local weather conditions. Domestic horses have been imported to nearly every continent, where their parasites are exposed to differing environments with varied climatic conditions. Regardless, certain common rules apply to understanding parasite ecology, which is the relationship of parasites to their environment. This chapter summarizes the effects of environmental factors on egg hatching, larval development, and survival of infective stages. A thorough comprehension of these principles will inform practitioners not only of *where* and *how* their patients become infected but, of equal importance, *when*. An expanded discussion of *refugia* will also increase the reader's understanding of the role of environmental stages in seasonal transmission, clinical disease, and genetic modifications of parasite populations over time.

Preparasitic development

For purposes of the following discussion, a distinction will be made between the development and persistence of preparasitic stages, particularly those of the strongyles. *Development* includes the processes of egg hatching and sequential progression through the first (L_1), second (L_2), and third (L_3) larval stages. In contrast, *persistence* refers to the duration of survival of L_3 stages in the environment. The chronology of free-living stages is illustrated in Figure 1.1.

Effects of temperature on development

Strongyle eggs generally hatch at temperatures above 7°C (43°F) and larval development occurs up to about 40°C (104°F). The optimum temperature for development of eggs and larvae is in the range 25–33°C (77–91°F), at which all developing larvae reach the infective L_3 stage within 3–4 days, with the highest larval yield at 28°C (82°F). No egg development is observed at temperatures below 4°C (39°F), while hatching requires 12–14 days at 6–10°C (43–50°F), 2–7 days at 10–20°C (50–70°F), 1–2 days at 20–30°C (70–86°F), and less than one day at 31–38°C (86–100°F) (Nielsen *et al.*, 2007).

Effects of freezing on development

Myths and misconceptions are common regarding the survival of free-living larval stages in freezing temperatures. The

Handbook of Equine Parasite Control, Second Edition. Martin K. Nielsen and Craig R. Reinemeyer.
© 2018 John Wiley & Sons, Inc. Published 2018 by John Wiley & Sons, Inc.

expression "killing frost" has been applied to insects and plants, and it is often erroneously assumed that it describes what happens to preparasitic nematodes as well. Although freezing can have detrimental effects on eggs and larvae on pasture, its total impact is sufficiently limited that the adjective "killing" is a misnomer under practical circumstances (Nielsen *et al.*, 2007).

The various free-living stages differ in their susceptibility to cold. Several laboratory studies have determined that long-term freezing damages strongyle eggs and reduces larval yield significantly. Unembryonated eggs appear to withstand frost better than embryonated eggs, while L_1 and L_2 larvae were most susceptible to freezing. Third stage larvae were generally the most resistant to cold. More than 90% of all L_1s and L_2s died after 1–4 days at −6 to −10 °C (21 to −14 °F) (Nielsen *et al.*, 2007).

To understand conditions in the field, it is also relevant to consider the effect of successive cycles of frost and thaw, which often occur during winter in temperate climates. Alternate freezing and thawing has a deleterious effect on most stages of strongyles, but unembryonated eggs were relatively unaffected by up to 97 days of occasional freeze/thaw cycles (Nielsen *et al.*, 2007). In comparison, embryonated eggs and first and second stage larvae succumbed under identical conditions. Regardless, freeze/thaw cycles can be mitigated completely by the effects of snow cover. A few centimeters of snow on the ground shelters the strongylid microenvironment and essentially maintains constant temperatures close to 0 °C (32 °F). Thus, snow cover is protective for unembryonated eggs and an intact fecal ball apparently provides additional security against fluctuating temperatures.

Effects of moisture on development

Moisture is another critical requirement for development of equine strongyle larvae. The lower limit for successful larval development appears to be 15–20% moisture in the feces and optimal fecal moisture content was determined to be 57–63%. One study found that L_1s survived for only a few days in feces that were rapidly desiccated (Ogbourne, 1972). In contrast, slower desiccation supported development to the L_2 stage, and a high percentage of those larvae survived and were capable of resuming development to L_3s when moisture was eventually supplemented (Nielsen *et al.*, 2007). Third stage larvae, in contrast, appear quite resistant to desiccation as long as they are protected by an intact fecal ball. This phenomenon can be explained by the metabolism and energy storage capabilities of preparasitic stages, which are described later in this chapter. In most climates, it is considered that the fecal ball does not desiccate fast enough to significantly inhibit development to the L_3 stage (Parnell, 1936; Uhlinger, 1991; Nielsen *et al.*, 2007).

Preparasitic persistence

Because persistence describes the duration of survival of third stage larvae in the environment, it also represents a measure of the risk of infection. The quantitative term for describing the numbers of third stage larvae on pasture is *infectivity*.

Energy reserves

In order to appreciate how third stage larvae survive the various environmental influences described previously, it is necessary to understand their energy metabolism and storage capabilities. Third stage larvae are surrounded by a protective membrane, which is the discarded sheath of the L_2 stage. This membrane completely surrounds the L_3, effectively preventing it from ingesting any nutrients (Figure 9.10). As a consequence, third stage larvae must survive solely on energy reserves stored in their intestinal cells in the form of lipids and carbohydrates. If these larvae are highly active, they quickly use up the energy reserves and expire if not ingested by a horse. However, if larvae are less active, they can survive much longer because they don't exhaust their limited energy reserves. Conditions that permit high larval activity include warm temperatures of 20–40 °C (70–104 °F) and high moisture levels or water films in which to move. In contrast, cold weather and/or desiccation restrict the movement of larvae, so they can survive for very long periods. Interestingly, larvae seem to resist even very hot weather if they remain in a desiccated state which doesn't allow mobility. In studies performed in Texas and tropical Australia, no larvae could be recovered from pasture herbage samples during dry periods, but subsequent rainfall allowed larvae to leave desiccated fecal balls and migrate on to the forage (Nielsen *et al.*, 2007). Moisture is a requirement for L3s to leave the fecal pat, so they can persist through longer periods of hot and dry weather if protected inside intact fecal balls.

Effects of temperature on persistence

Myths and misconceptions are common regarding the survival of free-living strongyle stages in freezing temperatures. Several laboratory studies have determined that L3s survived for longer intervals at 3 °C (37 °F) and −5 °C (23 °F) than at 31 °C (88 °F) and 26 °C (79 °F). Another study reported that freezing for 30 minutes or 72 hours had no effect on L3s, whereas constant freezing for five or eight months markedly reduced their survival (Nielsen *et al.*, 2007).

A proportion of L3s can tolerate alternating temperatures, but less than 1% survived five cycles of freezing for one to five days interrupted by thawing for a few

hours. The previous comments about the protective effects of snow cover apply to L3s as well, perhaps more so than to unembryonated eggs. When horses in northern temperate climates are turned out to spring pastures that haven't been grazed since the prior autumn, strongyle larvae will be out there waiting for them. Some larvae will have survived the entire winter as L3s, whereas others have developed recently from unembryonated eggs that were fortunate enough to find a protective microenvironment.

Effects of moisture on persistence

Moisture is also a critical factor in determining persistence of strongylid larvae. Larvae prefer to migrate in water films, and can only be mobile if there is sufficient moisture present in their microenvironment. It has been reported that strongyle larvae survived markedly better in intact versus disrupted fecal balls, and L3s kept on a glass slide survived desiccation in an incubator at 30 °C for 65 days.

Apparently, under certain temperature conditions, desiccation can protect rather than kill third stage larvae. Several reports document that L3s in a desiccated state withstand freezing better than larvae that were kept moist. One feasible explanation for these observations is the quantity and size of ice crystals formed during freezing. Ice crystals are capable of disrupting eggs and larvae at the cellular level, so it is logical that the combination of freezing and dry conditions would afford some protection.

Role of fecal balls

Fecal matter provides a highly protective habitat for eggs and larvae. When fecal balls remain intact, some moisture can be retained under the hardened surface and larvae are protected from ultraviolet irradiation, and somewhat from temperature fluctuations. These effects have been documented under field conditions in cold climates. The protective nature of intact feces supports the recommendation to spread manure (by harrowing, mowing or dragging pastures) at the end of the autumn grazing season if the pasture can be left unoccupied through winter. Long-term exposure of unprotected larvae to freezing temperatures or alternation between frost and thaw will most likely kill the majority before the following grazing season unless snow cover is nearly continuous.

The impact of various environmental factors on the individual, free-living stages of strongyle parasites is summarized in Table 3.1.

Computer simulations

The cumulative knowledge about the effects of temperature on cyathostomin larval development and persistence in the environment has recently been incorporated into a computer model (Leathwick, Donecker, and Nielsen, 2016). A set of outputs from this model is presented in Figure 3.1 to illustrate how quickly eggs hatch and larvae develop and how long each stage persists at different ranges of constant temperatures. In Figure 3.2, 10 years of climatic data from four different climatic regions were imported into the model, and the outputs illustrate the percent of cyathostomin eggs that successfully develop into L_3s through the course of the

Table 3.1 Effects of temperature on the survival, development, and persistence of free-living stages (eggs, L_1, L_2, L_3) of strongyles.

Development	Temperature range	Survival
No development above this level	>40 °C	Free-living stages die rapidly. Intact fecal balls may retain enough humidity to enable L_3 to survive for a shorter time period
Very rapid development to L_3 (often less than 1 day)	33–40 °C	L_3s will die quickly, but are able to survive for a few weeks inside intact fecal balls
Optimal temperature range for development of eggs and larvae. Larvae reach infective L_3 stage less than 4 days	25–33 °C	Larvae survive on the shorter term (*i.e.*, a few weeks), but conditions are too warm for long term survival
Eggs develop into L_3 in 2–3 weeks	10–25 °C	L_3 capable of surviving for several weeks to a few months
Lower limit for egg hatching is about 6 °C. Development to L_3 will take several weeks to a few months	6–10 °C	L_3 survive for many weeks and months
No hatching and no development	0–6 °C	Eggs and L_3 can survive for several months at temperatures just above the freezing point
No development during frost	<0 °C	Developing larvae (L_1 and L_2) are killed, but unembryonated eggs and L_3 can survive and persist for months, especially if protected by intact fecal balls and/or snow
Alternation between freezing and thawing will usually not lead to development unless temperatures exceed 6 °C	<0 > °C	Repeated freeze–thaw cycles are detrimental to egg and larval survival

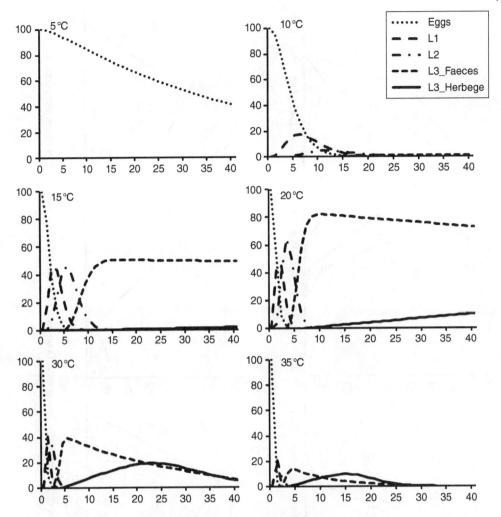

Figure 3.1 Model output showing the progression of development of strongyle eggs to L₃ larvae on pasture temperatures held at constant values of 5 °C, 10 °C, 15 °C, 20 °C, 30 °C, and 35 °C, and where no rainfall is allowed for. (*Source*: Reprinted from Veterinary Parasitology, 209, Leathwick, D.M., Donecker, J.M., and Nielsen, M.K., A model for the dynamics of the free-living states of equine cyathostomins, pp. 210–220, Copyright (2015), with permission from Elsevier).

year. This demonstrates that parasite transmission seasons are relatively brief in cold and northern temperate climates, whereas parasite transmission can take place during the majority of the year in warmer climates. It also shows that development can be quite variable between years.

Parasite refugia

The term *parasite refugia* has been introduced to explain some of the rather complex dynamics of anthelmintic resistance, which is discussed in Chapter 8. In simple terms, parasites within a defined population are considered to be *in refugia* when they are not exposed to a given drug at the time of anthelmintic treatment. Regardless of the treatment strategy and anthelmintic formulation chosen, only a portion of the target parasite population will be affected by the drug. Simplistically, the magnitude of this proportion affects the rate of resistance development over time, as it has a large impact on the selection pressure for resistant worms. In other

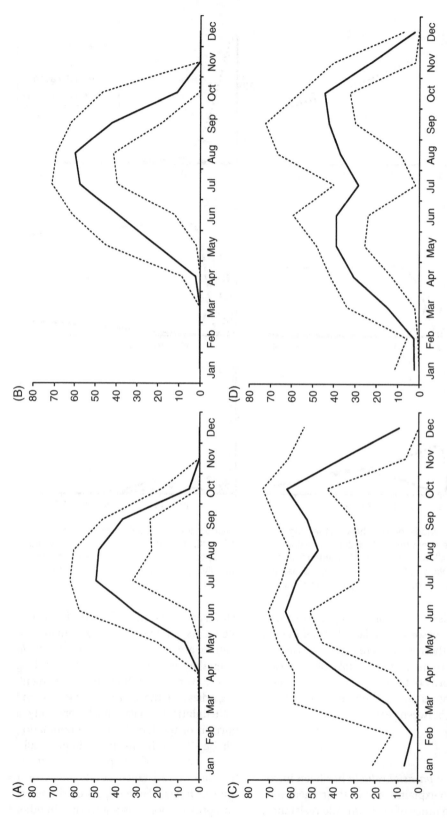

Figure 3.2 Model outputs showing the percent of strongyle eggs successfully developed to L$_3$ on pasture in four different climates: (A) northern temperate (South Dakota, USA), (B) temperate (Germany), (C) warm (Georgia, USA), and (D) hot (Texas, USA).

words, the parasites *in refugia* serve to dilute any resistant worms that may be accumulating in the population. This has been confirmed by experimental studies with sheep (Martin, Jambre, and Claxton, 1981; Dobson *et al.*, 2001, Waghorn *et al.*, 2008) as well as by computer modelling (Barnes, Dobson, and Barger, 1995; Leathwick, 2012).

As a practical example, consider a herd of horses grazing on pasture. They are all infected with cyathostomin nematodes. Some horses have larger burdens than others, but they all harbor some level of infection. A proportion of this cyathostomin population is comprised of adult worms in the large intestinal lumen, and another, larger proportion consists of encysted larval stages in the intestinal wall. A third proportion of the cyathostomin population consists of eggs and larvae on pasture. Depending on climate and season, the proportion of the entire parasite population that resides on pasture can be 90% or greater – by far the majority of the total community. Still, only a small proportion of these will be ingested by a horse and establish as parasites.

Essentially, there are two types of *refugia*. One could be called the *horse refugia* and the other could be termed *environmental refugia*. Horse *refugia* consist of parasitic stages that are not affected by an anthelmintic treatment. Obvious examples include encysted cyathostomin larvae during treatment with a non-larvicidal anthelmintic. Another example of horse *refugia* would be parasites in any herd members that are left untreated during implementation of a selective treatment strategy (see Chapter 7). Environmental *refugia* comprise all free-living (*i.e.*, preparasitic) stages on pasture or elsewhere in the environment.

The role of horse *refugia* will be covered elsewhere in this book (Chapters 7 and 8). Factors affecting environmental stages were covered previously in the present chapter.

It is important to understand that regardless of the life cycle phase (egg, larva, adult worm), the genes carried by individuals remain the same through the progression of stages. The entire environmental assemblage is derived from eggs passed by adult worms in the host, so both subpopulations share identical genotypic information.

Other parasites

Environmental conditions exert slightly different effects on the preparasitic stages of other equine parasites. A brief discussion of the more important parasites follows.

Parascaris spp.

Ascarids have a direct life cycle just like the strongyles, but achievement of infectivity does not require their eggs to hatch in the environment. Instead, horses are infected by ingesting embryonated eggs. Embryonated eggs persist quite well in deep litter, on surfaces in stalls, and on feeding equipment, and can even be recovered from the perineum and udder of mares. Ascarid eggs are additionally very resistant to most chemical disinfectants, including formalin and strong acids.

It is often claimed that embryonated ascarid eggs can remain infective in the environment for years, but these claims have not been substantiated in the scientific literature. Work with *Parascaris* eggs has illustrated that survival appears highly dependent on ambient temperature and soil type (Nielsen, 2016). One Swedish study found that the numbers of ascarid eggs in fecal piles placed on pasture and gravel plots were reduced by up to 50% over eight weeks during summer, but only by about 10% in plots contaminated during autumn (Lindgren *et al.*, 2009). Furthermore, eggs disappeared more quickly on well-drained gravel or sandy soils (Lindgren *et al.*, 2009). Interestingly, one study evaluating the effects of composting equine manure found that it took only 6–8 days of mean core temperatures of 35–55 °C to completely eliminate all *Parascaris* eggs (Gould *et al.*, 2013) from a compost pile. However, studies with swine ascarid eggs (*Ascaris suum*) have demonstrated that eggs can remain viable within the soil, so plowing pastures may provide only a temporary respite from ascarid infection. However, the benefit persists only until the pasture is plowed again in the future, when the eggs are returned to the soil surface, just as viable as before (Mejer, 2006).

Thus, available information suggests that eggs are unlikely to survive more than one year on pasture, unless they are protected from heat within intact fecal balls, deep litter, or by burial in the ground. However, it appears likely that equine ascarid eggs can overwinter if they are deposited relatively late in the season.

Therefore, foals born early in the following season are likely to pick up the overwintering infection, whereas foals born later in the year would be exposed to eggs passed in the same calendar year by older foals. Infection with *Parascaris* spp. can be described as a "foal-to-foal" disease, in which transmission occurs both within a given crop of foals and between crops of foals born in consecutive years.

Oxyuris equi

The maturation of *Oxyuris equi* eggs is ingeniously assisted by their use of the host as the "environmental site" of development. Deposition off eggs on the perineum ensures a dark, moist habitat with constant, warm temperatures and adequate oxygenation, at least for the few days the eggs require to larvate. Little is known about the environmental persistence of larvated pinworm eggs, but it is generally believed they can survive for several weeks. Human pinworm eggs (*Enterobius vermicularis*) have been shown to tolerate freezing, but they are more susceptible to warmer temperatures (Caldwell, 1982).

Tapeworms

All tapeworms have an indirect life cycle that features an intermediate host. The *Anoplocephala* and *Anoplocephaloides* species infecting horses use oribatid mites as intermediate hosts, and the horse becomes infected by accidentally ingesting the mites while grazing. Pasture infectivity, therefore, is essentially a function of mite populations and their ability to withstand various environmental factors. Numerous species of oribatid mites are known to serve as intermediate hosts for anoplocephalid cestodes, but relatively little is known about their epidemiology, so it is not possible to propose general rules for their longevity and infection rates. Although mites can survive cold winters to some extent, they are only active, and thus more available for ingestion, during the grazing season. Research has shown that the total numbers of oribatid mites on herbage correlates positively with temperature, relative humidity, rainfall and soil moisture (van Nieuwenhuizen *et al.*, 1994). As a consequence of increased mite exposure, tapeworm burdens tend to accumulate through the grazing season and peak during autumn in northern temperate climates. Regardless, given the ability of mites to survive winters, the potential for overwintering pasture infectivity of tapeworms is probably similar to that of strongyles and ascarids.

Conclusion

Generally speaking, the gastrointestinal parasites of horses have life cycles that are admirably adapted to recommence on an annual basis. Consequently, horse pastures are not expected to remain infective for more than one year, regardless of the geography, pasture type, or parasite category considered. Thus, potential infectivity doesn't accumulate during successive years. A horse pasture that has been grazed for 20 years contains no more strongylid larvae than one used for a single season.

References

Barnes, E.H., Dobson, R.J., and Barger, I.A. (1995) Worm control and anthelmintic resistance: Adventures with a model. *Parasitol. Today*, 11, 56–63.

Caldwell, J.P. (1982) Pinworms (*Enterobius vermicularis*). *Can. Fam. Phys.*, 28, 306–309.

Gould, J.C., Rossano, M.G., Lawrence, L.M., *et al.* (2013) The effects of windrow composting on the viability of *Parascaris equorum* eggs. *Vet. Parasitol.*, 191, 73–80.

Leathwick, D.M. (2012) Modelling the benefits of a new class of anthelmintic in combination. *Vet. Parasitol.*, 186, 93–100.

Leathwick, D.M., Donecker, J.M., and Nielsen, M.K. (2016) A model for the development and growth of the parasitic stages of *Parascaris* spp. in the horse. *Vet. Parasitol.*, 228, 108–115.

Lindgren, K.I.N., Roepstorff, A., Lind, E.O., and Höglund, J. (2009) Seasonal variation in development and survival of *Parascaris equorum* eggs in pasture or on gravel surface. *World Association for the Advancement of Veterinary Parasitology Conference*, Calgary, Canada, p. 36.

Martin, P.J., Le Jambre, L.F., and Claxton, J.H. (1981) The impact of *refugia* on the development of thiabendazole resistance in *Haemonchus contortus*. *Int. J. Parasitol.*, 11, 35–41.

Mejer, H. (2006) Transmission, infection dynamics and alternative control of helminths in organic swine. PhD thesis, The Royal Veterinary and Agricultural University, Samfundslitteratur Grafik, Copenhagen, Denmark.

Nielsen, M.K. (2016) Evidence-based considerations for control of *Parascaris* spp. infections in horses. *Equine Vet. Educ.*, 28, 224–231.

Nielsen, M.K., Kaplan, R.M., Thamsborg, S.M., *et al.* (2007) Climatic influences on development and survival of free-living stages of equine strongyles: Implications for worm control strategies and managing anthelmintic resistance. *Vet. J.*, 174, 23–32.

Ogbourne, C.P. (1972) Observations on the free-living stages of strongylid nematodes of horses. *Parasitology*, 64, 461–477.

Parnell, I.W. (1936) Notes on the survival of the eggs and free-living larvae of sclerostomes on pasture. *Sci. Agric.*, 16, 391–397.

Uhlinger, C.A. (1991) Equine small strongyles: epidemiology, pathology, and control. *Comp. Equine*, 13, 863–869.

van Nieuwenhuizen, L.C., Verster, A.J.M., Horak, I.G., *et al.* (1994) The seasonal abundance of oribatid mites (Acari: Cryptostigmata) on an irrigated Kikuyu grass pasture. *Exp. Appl. Acarol.*, 18, 73–86.

Waghorn, T.S., Leathwick, D.M., Miller, C.M., and Atkinson, D.S. (2008) Brave or gullible: Testing the concept that leaving susceptible parasites in *refugia* will slow the development of anthelmintic resistance. *N.Z. Vet. J.*, 56, 158–163.

4

Host Factors Affecting Parasite Transmission

Every host–parasite relationship involves countless interactions that affect transmission. These range from mortal combat to apparent collaborations, and occur from the molecular to the population level. In a successful and sustainable relationship, the host provides shelter and sustenance so a resident population of worms can reproduce and the tenants refrain from destroying their domicile. Vandalism is optional.

In any population of grazing horses, the distribution of parasites among the members of a herd will always be non-uniform and skewed. Some individuals will have large worm burdens, whereas the majority harbor small or moderate numbers. This pattern is often referred to as the 20/80 rule, meaning that 20% of the horses harbor 80% of the parasites in any given herd. The same general pattern is observed in the levels of strongyle egg shedding within an equine population (Kaplan and Nielsen, 2010). As a consequence, problematic strongyle transmission is always caused by a minority of the horses in a group. Understanding these egg-shedding patterns is the key to monitoring and controlling parasite transmission in certain individuals for the mutual benefit of the entire community. The reasons why some horses shed high numbers of eggs and others very low numbers are not well understood, but a few factors can be identified with certainty.

Immunity

Host immunity plays a major role in limiting the transmission of nearly all parasitisms, but equids host two examples that are unique among grazing animals for their near totality: *Parascaris* spp. and *Strongyloides westeri*. It is uncommon and rare, respectively, to encounter adult horses with patent infections of these nematodes. In comparison, horses of all ages can be infected with cyathostomins and *A. perfoliata*. Current knowledge about the role of the equine immune system in regulating important equine parasitisms is summarized herein.

Large strongyles

Horses develop a relatively strong immune response to infection with *S. vulgaris*, and attempts to immunize horses with irradiated infective larvae were quite successful (Klei *et al.*, 1982; Monahan *et al.*, 1994) under conditions of artificial infection. Observations made by both authors further suggest that untreated foals, weanling, and yearlings generally harbour greater numbers of *S. vulgaris* specimens than mature horses from the same herd. It appears that migration within the arterial circulation affords sufficient, direct exposure of parasite antigens to the host immune system to elicit an effective response. It remains unknown whether other *Strongylus* species

Handbook of Equine Parasite Control, Second Edition. Martin K. Nielsen and Craig R. Reinemeyer.
© 2018 John Wiley & Sons, Inc. Published 2018 by John Wiley & Sons, Inc.

can elicit similar immune responses, but it is certainly possible.

Cyathostomins

Immunity has been observed to play a rather sophisticated role in regulating the dynamics and progression of cyathostomin infections through the various larval stages to adulthood. Readers are referred to Chapter 1 for a complete description of the life cycle. Summarized briefly, the incoming third stage larvae burrow into the mucosal walls of the large intestine, where they go through the early and late L_3 stage and progress to L_4 before they emerge into the lumen of the intestine. Larvae can undergo arrested development at the early third larval stage (EL_3) and amass huge numbers of encysted stages in the large intestine.

In foals, ingested cyathostomin larvae apparently progress steadily through all larval stages without becoming arrested (Nielsen and Lyons, 2017). Similarly, another study found that yearlings had lower encysted proportions compared to 2 to 5 year olds (Chapman, French, and Klei, 2003). In contrast, yearlings had higher numbers of adult parasites compared to their older pasture mates. Furthermore, encysted cyathostomin burdens were observed to accumulate over the grazing season to reach their peaks in autumn. Taken together, this can be interpreted as an effect of the host immune response to the incoming L_3s. Foals and yearlings have not yet mounted an immune response to cyathostomin infection, which can explain why arrested development does not appear to occur. It should be noted that EL_3 numbers typically exceed those of later stages by substantial margins, which suggests that a large proportion of EL_3s are killed by the host response and never make it to adulthood. Parasite factors play a role as well and will be described in Chapter 5.

Observational studies have demonstrated that strongyle worm burdens tend to remain fairly constant in horses as they age, but the corresponding egg counts decline chronologically (Chapman, French, and Klei, 2003). This suggests that the main effect of immunity is not to prevent parasite establishment but rather to control the fecundity of female worms and thereby affect transmission.

Other studies have shown that intensive anthelmintic treatment of horses through one grazing season made them more susceptible to challenge infections during the following year (Monahan *et al.*, 1997). These findings support the notion that acquired immunity has an operative role in parasite transmission, although horses never become completely immune to strongyles.

Additional observations suggest that certain innate mechanisms may also help the host to regulate transmission. For example, the magnitude of strongyle egg shedding by adult horses is strikingly consistent over time and is particularly stable in horses that pass low numbers of strongyle eggs (*i.e.*, <200 EPG) (Nielsen, Haaning, and Olsen, 2006; Becher *et al.*, 2010). The effector mechanisms of this phenomenon remain unclear, but a genetic component is likely to be involved. If so, it is expected that various blood lines within a breed would exhibit patterns of egg shedding that differ significantly from the norm. This hypothesis is supported by findings in ruminants, where resilience to parasite infection has been shown to be hereditary (Stear *et al.*, 1984; Gasbarre, Leighton, and Davies, 1990). Recently, a comprehensive study evaluated the repeatability and heritability of fecal egg counts in 789 pure-blood Arabian horses (Kornaś *et al.*, 2015). The authors found low repeatability of strongyle fecal egg counts across the eight study years and that only 10% of the observed egg count variation had a genetic origin.

However, horses over three years of age had substantially higher heritability estimates (21%), which suggest that genetic regulation of egg count levels could be related to development of immunity.

Parascaris spp.

As previously mentioned, ascarid infection invokes a strong immune response. This immunity has been found to be primarily age-dependent, *i.e.*, it occurs even in the total absence of ascarid exposure (Leathwick, Donecker, and Nielsen, 2016). However, there is some evidence of acquired immunity as well because worm burdens were observed to diminish in foals vaccinated with large priming doses of irradiated *Parascaris* eggs (Bello, 1985). Observations suggest that the chronology of events following the onset of the immune response to *Parascaris* spp. is as follows: (1) reduction of egg shedding, (2) expulsion of adult worms, and (3) expulsion of a second wave of infection, if present. Adult worms can be found within the intestines of 5 to 6 month old foals, even after egg counts were observed to decrease. This is consistent with observations that ascarid egg counts decline before adult ascarid burdens disappear, as demonstrated ultrasonically (Nielsen *et al.*, 2016). Similar to cyathostomins, the immature (L_4) stages or *Parascaris* spp. are more numerous than adult parasites (Fabiani, Lyons, and Nielsen, 2016), and this appears to occur with both the first and the second waves of infection. Taken together, this suggests that a large proportion of the larvae are killed before they can mature and reproduce.

Tapeworms

The limited information available suggests a minor host immune response to infection with *A. perfoliata*. Infection intensity does not appear to be age-related, but rather is associated with access to pasture, where infections are acquired while grazing. Interestingly, among the parasite categories discussed herein, the equine tapeworm is the least invasive and never leaves the intestinal tract, whereas large strongyles and ascarids all have migratory phases, and cyathostomins spend considerable intervals encysted within host tissues. It is feasible that cumulative tissue contact helps to stimulate an immune response.

Grazing behavior

Pastures grazed by horses develop a distinct pattern of usage, characterized by areas known as "roughs" and "lawns". Roughs consist of large or small islets of unconsumed forage, and are areas of pasture where horses defecate but do not graze. In contrast, lawns are areas where horses graze, but do not defecate. The herbage of lawns can become quite short in over-stocked pastures. Horses have an aversion for ingesting forage in proximity to fecal deposits, so these spatial patterns develop as a consequence of fecal avoidance behavior. Grazing cattle behave similarly, although unconsumed forage is distributed focally rather than organized into large areas. In all grazing animals, fecal avoidance behaviour is apparently driven by the sense of smell (Hansen, 1982).

The numbers of infective strongyle larvae in roughs have been shown to be 10 to 15 times higher than in lawns (Herd and Willardson, 1985). Thus, selective grazing behavior provides an elegant, natural system by which horses may regulate their parasite exposure. As long as pastures are not overgrazed, resident horses can continue to eschew the roughs, thereby diminishing their daily intake of infective larvae. On a pasture with limited herbage, however, pecking order dynamics may force the lowest-ranking individuals to graze farther into the roughs. Thus, horses grazing the same pasture can have dis-similar parasite exposures, and their resulting parasite burdens are expected to be different. This circumstance may explain, in part, the skewed distribution of parasite populations within a herd of horses.

Stress

The impact of stress on host immunity is well-documented (Segerstrom and Miller, 2004), although the component mechanisms are highly complex and the physiologic effects can be very difficult to measure. Relevant to the current discussion, strongyle egg counts routinely increase in response to host stress, and demonstration thereof requires no specialized equipment or training (see Chapter 9).

Field observations by one of the authors (MKN) suggest that new arrivals to a farm are likely to have significantly higher strongyle egg counts than permanent residents. The multiple stressors that accompany transfer include adjustment to new premises and diet, interacting with a different microbiotic environment, and establishment within the social dominance hierarchy. The effects of transport and translocation on strongyle egg counts need to be confirmed in larger studies.

Case records from equine referral hospitals often indicate that their patient populations exhibit high strongyle egg counts. In comparison to recent herd records for the same individual, a health condition requiring hospital admission may be accompanied by a 10-fold or greater increase in egg counts. Because this expansion occurs over a relatively short time period, it can be assumed that adult worm burdens are relatively unchanged. Thus, the only feasible explanation is increased fecundity of female worms. Stress, therefore, may not affect the size of the worm burden in the short term, but rather the magnitude of egg shedding.

Athletic competition is another well-known source of equine stress because it requires strenuous training and frequent transportation to competitive events. In one pertinent example, Standardbred Trotters that had more racing success during a single season exhibited a tendency toward higher strongyle egg counts compared to the remainder of "also-rans" (Fog, Vigre, and Nielsen, 2011). The performance of winning horses was obviously not impeded by their worm burdens, but the accompanying stress putatively contributed to increased egg output and thus potentiated parasite transmission.

Physiologic stress is accompanied by temporary or sustained elevations of plasma cortisol. Equine Cushing's disease (pituitary *pars intermedia* dysfunction) is a common endocrine disease of middle-aged to geriatric horses, which is characterized by excess secretion of adrenocorticotropic hormone and increased production of corticosteroid hormones by the adrenal gland. One recent study reported that horses with Cushing's disease had significantly higher strongyle egg counts than age-matched controls (McFarlane *et al.*, 2010). It is possible that Cushing's horses have larger worm burdens, but it is more likely that their compromised immune function allows resident parasites to shed higher numbers of eggs *per capita*.

Similarly, it is often assumed that geriatric horses (aged 20 years and older) require more intensive parasite control efforts. Any horse may begin to shed higher numbers of strongyle eggs if it experiences dental problems or loses body condition, and these health issues are more common in aged horses. Although some studies reported higher egg counts in horses ≥20 years (Döpfer *et al.*, 2004; Adams *et al.*, 2015), another epidemiologic survey observed no differences in this age group (Osterman Lind *et al.*, 1999). In general, the egg counts of healthy, geriatric horses in good body condition should be monitored for possible increases with increasing age.

In addition to these examples, studies in non-equid host species have demonstrated that concurrent infection with other infectious agents can lead to higher worm burdens and higher levels of egg shedding (Supali *et al.*, 2010). Thus, parasite burdens might require extra attention in horses with concurrent illnesses.

Concluding remarks

Although the mechanisms that regulate parasite transmission are not fully understood, we can at least identify horses that require more anthelmintic treatments than others. It is well known that younger horses always need more attention in parasite control programs. However, in order to control parasite transmission more effectively, it is equally important to consider new arrivals, horses that are subordinate in the herd hierarchy, competitive horses being transported frequently to events, and horses that are unhealthy due to non-parasitic causes. Egg-shedding patterns almost always follow the 20/80 rule, and even in the absence of the above-mentioned risk factors, there will always be a few high-shedding horses in every herd. It is therefore important to identify this high-contaminating minority for optimal management of the entire group.

References

Adams, A.A., Betancourt, A., Barker, V.D., *et al.* (2015) Comparison of the immunologic response to anthelmintic treatment in old versus middle-aged horses. *J. Equine Vet. Sci.*, 35, 873–881.

Becher, A., Mahling, M., Nielsen, M.K., and Pfister, K. (2010) Selective anthelmintic therapy of horses in the Federal States of Bavaria (Germany) and Salzburg (Austria): An investigation into strongyle egg shedding consistency. *Vet. Parasitol.*, 171, 116–122.

Bello, T.R. (1985) The insidious invasive verminous antigens of the horse. *J. Equine Vet. Sci.*, 5, 163–167.

Chapman, M.R., French, D.D., and Klei, T.R. (2003) Prevalence of strongyle nematodes in naturally infected ponies of different ages and during different seasons of the year in Louisiana. *J. Parasitol.*, 89, 309–314.

Döpfer, D., Kerssens, C.M., Meijer, Y.G., *et al.* (2004) Shedding consistency of strongyle-type eggs in Dutch boarding horses. *Vet. Parasitol.*, 124, 249–258.

Fabiani, J.V., Lyons, E.T., and Nielsen, M.K. (2016) Dynamics of *Parascaris* and *Strongylus* spp. parasites in untreated juvenile horses. *Vet. Parasitol.*, 30, 62–66.

Fog, P., Vigre, H., and Nielsen, M.K. (2011) Strongyle egg counts in Standardbred trotters: Are they associated with race performance? *Equine Vet. J.*, 43, 89–92.

Gasbarre, L.C., Leighton, E.A., and Davies, C.J. (1990) Genetic control of immunity to gastrointestinal nematodes of cattle. *Vet. Parasitol.*, 37, 267–272.

Hansen, J.W. (1982) The influence of stocking rate on the uptake of trichostrongyle larvae. PhD Thesis. Royal Veterinary and Agricultural University, Copenhagen, Denmark.

Herd, R.P. and Willardson, K.L. (1985) Seasonal distribution of infective strongyle larvae on horse pastures. *Equine Vet. J.*, 17, 235–237.

Kaplan, R.M. and Nielsen, M.K. (2010) An evidence-based approach to equine parasite control: It ain't the 60s anymore. *Equine Vet. Educ.*, 22, 306–316.

Klei, T.R., Torbert, B.J., Chapman, M.R., and Ochoa, R. (1982) Irradiated larval vaccination of ponies against *Strongylus vulgaris*. *J. Parasitol.*, 68, 561–569.

Kornaś, S., Sallé, G., Skalska, M., *et al.* (2015) Estimation of genetic parameters for resistance to gastro-intestinal nematodes in pure blood Arabian horses. *Int. J. Parasitol.*, 45, 237–242.

Leathwick, D.M., Donecker, J.M., and Nielsen, M.K. (2016) A model for the development and growth of the parasitic stages of *Parascaris* spp. in the horse. *Vet. Parasitol.*, 228, 108–115.

McFarlane, D., Hale, G.M., Johnson, E.M., and Maxwell, L.K. (2010) Fecal egg counts after anthelmintic administration to aged horses and horses with pituitary pars intermedia dysfunction. *J. Am. Vet. Med. Assoc.*, 236, 330–334.

Monahan, C.M., Taylor, H.W., Chapman, M.R., and Klei, T.R. (1994) Experimental immunization of ponies with *Strongylus vulgaris* radiation-attenuated larvae or crude soluble somatic extracts from larval or adult stages. *J. Parasitol.*, 80, 911–923.

Monahan, C.M., Chapman, M.R., Taylor, H.W., *et al.* (1997) Foals raised on pasture with or without daily pyrantel tartrate feed additive: Comparison of parasite burdens and host responses following experimental challenge with large and small strongyle larvae. *Vet. Parasitol.*, 73, 277–289.

Nielsen, M.K. and Lyons, E.T. (2017) Encysted cyathostomin larvae in foals – progression of stages and the effect of seasonality. *Vet. Parasitol.*, 236, 108–112.

Nielsen, M.K., Haaning, N., and Olsen, S.N. (2006) Strongyle egg shedding consistency in horses on farms using selective therapy in Denmark. *Vet. Parasitol.*, 135, 333–335.

Nielsen, M.K., Donoghue, E.M., Stephens, M.L., *et al.* (2016) An ultrasonographic scoring method for transabdominal monitoring of ascarid burdens in foals. *Equine Vet. J.*, 48, 380–386.

Osterman Lind, E., Höglund, J., Ljungström, B.L., *et al.* (1999) A field survey on the distribution of strongyle infections of horses in Sweden and factors affecting faecal egg counts. *Equine Vet. J.*, 31, 68–72.

Segerstrom, S.C. and Miller, G.E. (2004) Psychological stress and the human immune system: A meta-analytic study of 30 years of inquiry. *Psychol. Bull.*, 130, 601–630.

Stear, M.J., Nicholas, F.W., Brown, S.C., *et al.* (1984) The relationship between the bovine major histocompatibility system and faecal worm egg counts, in *Immunogenetic Approaches to the Control of Endoparasites* (eds J.K. Dineen and P.M. Outteridge), Division of Animal Health, CSIRO, Melbourne, pp. 126–133.

Supali, T., Verweij, J.J., Wiria, A.E., *et al.* (2010) Polyparasitism and its impact on the immune system. *Int. J. Parasitol.*, 40, 1171–1176.

5

Parasite Factors Affecting Parasite Transmission

Most parasites could be thought of as reincarnated, 17 year old boys. Their major interests in life are eating and sex, and not necessarily in that order. In physical form, most nematodes are little more than a cylindrical package of reproductive organs. The digestive tract is a simple tube, so even the basic organs of life support are reduced to a minimum. Egg production is the most critical factor in life for these invertebrates, and all necessary resources are diverted to that purpose. Apropos to this strategy, female nematodes are often two or more times the size of their male counterparts.

A central tenet of biology is that success for any organism can be defined as propagation of the next generation. To achieve such success, biological organisms must constantly evolve to adapt to changing environments. Even the simplest parasitic helminths of veterinary interest occupy at least two different habitats during a typical life cycle: the vertebrate host and the external environment, where transmission occurs. In comparison to feral host populations, the forces of change are many times greater for parasites in domesticated animals because numerous management factors (*e.g.*, diet, hygiene, confinement versus turnout, use of anthelmintics) can alter both the host and the environment in terms of parasite survival and reproduction.

This chapter will review some of the parasite factors that affect transmission, *i.e.*, successful propagation of the next generation.

Reproduction

Fecundity

A basic survival strategy of many parasitic species is to overwhelm the odds against success by sheer force of numbers. If only 1% of the eggs of a particular species manage to develop into a subsequent generation, the odds of survival are obviously greater if many, many eggs are produced.

Fecundity is defined as the average number of reproductive products produced per unit of time by a single female organism. The females of some parasitic species are extremely fecund, and the Ascaridoid nematodes are widely considered the champions of this strategy. For example, the ascarid of humans, *Ascaris lumbricoides*, is estimated to produce approximately 200,000 eggs per day (Sinniah, 1982). The egg-producing capacity of *Parascaris* spp. has not been estimated, but it is likely to be of similar magnitude.

Reliable figures are not available for the average fecundity of other parasites, such as large or small strongyles. Some sources report that adult female pinworms can produce 60,000 eggs in a single event (Reinemeyer and Nielsen, 2014). However, since the adult females often expire after this supreme effort, oviposition by pinworms may be a one-time event.

Members of the subclass Strongylinae (large strongyles) tend to be larger, on average, and are thus likely more fecund than

Handbook of Equine Parasite Control, Second Edition. Martin K. Nielsen and Craig R. Reinemeyer.
© 2018 John Wiley & Sons, Inc. Published 2018 by John Wiley & Sons, Inc.

most genera that comprise the Cyathostominae. One study enumerated the numbers of eggs found in the uteri of specimens of equine strongylid species and found that counts varied from fewer than 50 in some of the smaller cyathostomins to several thousand in a large strongyle such as *S. edentatus* (Kuzmina *et al.*, 2012). However, the rate at which eggs are released may vary considerably, so fecundity may not be a simple function of worm size. Illustrating this point, the aforementioned study also found an inverse relationship between abundance of a given parasite within the population studied and its egg capacity (Kuzmina *et al.*, 2012). In other words, species that were present in very high numbers were harboring relatively few eggs per worm, whereas species of lower intensity contained a higher number of eggs per female. This is completely logical from a biological perspective, as a highly abundant parasite has an interest in increasing genetic diversity by allowing contributions from as many individuals as possible. The critical goal for a less abundant species, in contrast, is merely to survive, *i.e.*, to ensure that at least some representatives can form a new generation. This intricate inter-regulation of egg shedding is perhaps the main explanation for an apparent lack of a direct correlation between egg counts and worm numbers (see Chapter 9 for further reading).

Translation

Translation is defined as the series of changes undergone by a reproductive product (*e.g.*, egg, larva) to render it infective to a host. This definition is similar to that of development, but the latter term can be used to discuss changes from one stage to another. In contrast, translation refers to the entire itinerary, from the stage that leaves one host to the stage that infects another. As an example, freshly passed strongylid eggs are not directly infective to their definitive hosts; the eggs must first hatch and develop progressively to the infective, third stage (L_3). For the common parasites of horses, most of this development takes place in the environment, as discussed in greater detail in Chapter 3. During that process, life cycle stages are subjected to the vagaries of the indigenous climate. One notable exception is the equine pinworm, *Oxyuris equi*, which attaches its eggs to the skin of the host's perianal area. For several days thereafter, the body temperature of the host provides a well-controlled habitat in which the eggs rapidly become infective. The tail-rubbing behavior often elicited by this parasite subsequently serves as an elegant catalyst for contaminating the horse's environment. Through this adaptation, pinworm eggs are able to translate more quickly and with a higher rate of success than if left totally to environmental influences.

Persistence of infective stages

The ultimate strategy of a parasite is to introduce an infective stage into the body of the definitive host through the preferred, proven route. The odds of success increase significantly if infective stages can be presented to the host over a prolonged period of time. Thus, those parasites with extremely persistent infective stages have an evolutionary advantage for successful parasitism. The documented persistence of infective stages of the common equine helminths ranges from weeks to months, with marked variation determined by climatic conditions.

Transmission

Transmission is the entrance of an infective stage into the body of the intended host. Most helminth parasites of equids are transmitted via inadvertent ingestion, which is an appropriate strategy for a definitive host that is an obligate grazer. Parasitic infection is admittedly a haphazard consequence of the grazing lifestyle, but some parasites have adapted specific strategies to increase the likelihood of transmission.

One example is the proteinaceous coating of *Parascaris* eggs. This covering helps to protect eggs from environmental conditions, but it may also enhance their ability to adhere to fomites in the environment, including the vertical walls of stalls, and the udder of a mare. The latter site virtually ensures infection of foals during the process of suckling and the former exploits the characteristic behavior of foals to explore their environs orally. Similarly, the passage of *Oxyuris equi* eggs in clumps virtually ensures that any accidental encounter by a susceptible host will result in multiple, simultaneous exposures.

Adult *Gasterophilus* flies attach their eggs to specific sites on the haircoat of the horse. Some species deposit their eggs in a location from which they can migrate into the oral cavity. For example, *G. nasalis* oviposits in the intermandibular area and hatching first instars make their way through the commissures of the lips and into the mouth. Other bot species lay their eggs in locations that are accessible to oral ingestion by the host or herd mates; oviposition by *G. intestinalis* females on the lower limbs is a well-known example. Grooming by the horse (specifically, the carbon dioxide content and high humidity of exhaled air cause eggs to hatch) facilitates direct introduction of first instars into the oral cavity. However, *G. intestinalis* eggs are often deposited on the mane and withers as well, areas that clearly cannot be reached by the primary host. However, mutual grooming by herd mates targets these specific areas, so the instars are successfully transferred to an equid host, albeit not the one on which the eggs were initially deposited.

Another exceptional adaptation for transmission is seen in *Strongyloides westeri*, which can maintain a free-living life cycle for several generations in the total absence of equid hosts. The lactogenic route of transmission represents an additional, unique adaptation that allows *Strongyloides* to be the first parasite to infect the intestinal tract of a foal. *Strongyloides* is also unique in that infection may be acquired percutaneously, so oral ingestion is not required.

Filarioid nematodes live within tissues or occupy host sites that have no direct connection with the external environment, so transmission is problematic. However, most filarioids exploit hematophagous arthropods as a means for escaping the host, and also as the preferred site for essential development in the environment. Thus, *Onchocerca* microfilariae migrate to the skin, where they are ingested by certain biting flies. These arthropods nurture all the essential stages of translation and ultimately transfer the nematode into a new host via their feeding activities.

Finally, the parasitologic literature reports many examples of intermediate hosts whose behavior is modified by the infective parasitic stages that they harbor (Chubb, Ball, and Parker, 2009). Such altered behaviors inevitably increase the likelihood that the intermediate host will be consumed by a definitive host, thus promoting propagation of the next parasitic generation. All cestode parasites of horses are transmitted through ingestion of soil mites of the family Oribatidae. Oribatid mites are mobile, but there is no evidence that the behavior of mites infected with cysticercoids is altered in any fashion that would ultimately favor parasitic transmission.

Propagation of life cycle stages

As mentioned in Chapter 4, the regulation of the cyathostomin life cycle is a complex phenomenon involving host, environmental, and parasitic factors. Arrested development of the EL_3 stage is believed to be triggered by three main factors: the host immune response, pre-conditioning of environmental stages by climatic conditions, and repressive signals from the population of adult parasites occupying the intestinal lumen. The messengers and pathways of these parasitic signals have not yet been identified.

Persistence of adult parasites

The scientific literature contains remarkably little information about the longevity of various internal parasite species. Prior to the application of radiolabeled molecules, it was impossible to track the fate of individual worms within a population. It is even problematic to monitor the characteristics of an entire population unless the host is maintained under circumstances that obviate reinfection.

There is little advantage for a parasite to hang around once it has accomplished its major objective and contributed to the propagation of a new generation. Accordingly, most species demonstrate a spike in reproductive activity soon after reaching maturity, and egg laying diminishes steadily thereafter over time. The inevitable decline in fecundity may be due to senescence of the parasite, but host immunity also serves to limit egg production in some host/parasite systems.

From an evolutionary standpoint, it would make sense for parasites to maintain maximal reproductive activity throughout any season in which the environmental conditions for translation and transmission are favorable. In most climates, the maximum duration would be approximately 6 months, but few species maintain peak reproductive activity for such a long interval.

In general, none of the common equine intestinal parasites survive as adults within the horse for more than one year.

Furthermore, worm burdens are not increased through the accumulation of subsequent generations. A young adult cyathostomin would rarely encounter one of its parents while wandering around the neighborhood, let alone its grandmother. Rather, luminal parasite populations are replaced at least once annually, and their life cycles all appear well adapted to the calendar year.

Examples

The average lifespan for adult large strongyles and cyathostomins after achieving maturity is probably no more than 3 to 4 months (Reinemeyer *et al.*, 1986). Adult strongyles are present in the intestinal lumen throughout winter, and they do yield some level of contamination with eggs that face a rather bleak future. Perhaps the major purpose of adult persistence is to keep that niche occupied, thereby "holding" larval stages in mucosal tissues until environmental conditions are more favorable for translation.

Bot flies (*Gasterophilus* spp.) are all considered univoltine, meaning they develop only a single generation annually. Of that interval, they spend only a few days as adults, approximately one month as eggs, and the remainder as first through third larval instars or pupae.

Little is known about the longevity of equine cestodes, but tapeworms can be some of the most long-lived creatures in the helminth pantheon. It is likely that individual cestodes that are acquired during the grazing season are able to survive through winter and at least until the beginning of the subsequent grazing cycle. Thus, the evidence suggests that the tapeworm lifespan is no more than one year and that the life cycle is adapted to an annual cycle, similar to the strongyles.

Adult filarioids are known to survive for several years in the tissues of the definitive host. *Onchocerca* apparently exhibits this characteristic because dermatologic signs caused by microfilariae tend to recur annually.

Seasonality of reproduction

One thing that distinguishes helminth parasites from other infectious organisms is the requirement for reproductive products to return to the environment (*i.e.*, outside the host) where they must undergo some essential change before becoming infective to another host. Thus, it is only logical that equine parasites would have evolved to exploit these environmental limitations to the fullest. The single best example of this exploitation is synchronization of their reproductive activities (*i.e.*, egg laying) with the seasonality of environmental conditions that are suitable for translation and transmission.

Ascarids

Ascarid infection patterns have a pronounced seasonality, but this appears to be mostly driven by foal age and, hence, immune status. Climatic influences may play some role, but it is likely to be less pronounced than for other parasite categories. Seasonality is determined by the fact that most foals are born in late winter and spring. These foals will be exposed to infective ascarid eggs present in the environment since the prior year, and infections are established quickly. By about 5 months of age, both ascarid worm burdens and egg counts reach their peak, after which they quickly decline as the foals begin mounting an immune response (Fabiani, Lyons, and Nielsen, 2016). Depending on when the foals were born, this peak contamination of the environment happens during summer or early autumn. An unknown proportion of these eggs will persist through winter to infect the coming year's foal crop.

Large strongyles

The acquisition of larval infections during the grazing season, combined with the protracted prepatent periods of the large strongyles, result in the onset of patency several months later, typically near the start of a new grazing season. The long PPP of large strongyles may have been an evolutionary adaptation to inefficient reproductive activities (*e.g.*, producing eggs that end up in a snow drift). A PPP that extends through winter neatly allows patency to be synchronized with climatic conditions that are favorable for egg hatching and development of larvae.

From the standpoint of practical control, the prolonged life cycles of large strongyles make them particularly susceptible to control efforts. This will be covered in greater detail in Chapters 7 and 12.

Cyathostomins

The life cycles of cyathostomins, at least those that develop progressively, are much shorter than those of the large strongyles. When arrested development is implemented, however, their total times of residence might be two to three times longer. New larval infections are acquired during the grazing season, and a portion of the newly acquired larvae mature quickly and begin to lay eggs later in the same grazing season. This population may be responsible for the so-called "summer rise" of strongylid egg counts reported by Herd in 1986. However, other members of the population might undergo prolonged arrested development as early third stage larvae (EL$_3$s) in the mucosa of the cecum or ventral colon. Eventually they develop to the late third (LL$_3$) and fourth larval stages (L$_4$) within fibrous cysts in the gut mucosa, and total residence in the host before maturity may exceed two years (Gibson, 1953).

Ultimately, worms emerge from the mucosal cysts and begin to reproduce; this often occurs in synchrony with the onset of the local grazing season. Thus, in northern temperate climates, we see the so-called "spring rise" in strongylid egg counts during March to May (Poynter, 1954; Duncan, 1974). This phenomenon serves to contaminate the environment just when environmental conditions virtually ensure successful translation of infective larvae. In feral, free-ranging herds, this also coincides with the availability of non-immune, susceptible juveniles that are beginning to practice grazing as an essential means of acquiring nutrients.

The prolonged arrested development of cyathostomes within gut tissues is unparalleled among nematode parasites of domestic animals. Certain nematodes can become arrested in various somatic tissues, such as *Toxocara canis* or *Ancylostoma caninum* in visceral tissues of dogs, *Trichinella spiralis* in the muscle tissues of virtually any intermediate host, and even *Strongyloides westeri* in the ventral abdominal wall of a mare. However, no other species, let alone an entire subfamily, has arrested stages that remain in the bowel for longer than a single annual cycle. The persistence of populations in arrested development for greater than two grazing seasons must be a response to certain evolutionary pressures, but the exact nature of those selection factors remains speculative. Such an adaptation would be logical if environmental conditions favorable for translation were ephemeral or even absent in selected habitats. It would also make sense if prehistoric equids were nomadic, but returned to preferred grazing areas at intervals that were greater than once annually. Since larvae in the environment generally cannot survive for much longer than one year, prolonged arrest provides a mechanism by which vital, reproducing populations could be ensured, and eggs for environmental contamination would be available to infect the new pasturage to facilitate transmission within just a few weeks.

It should be noted here that encysted stages of cyathostomins are not uniformly susceptible to any anthelmintic regimen, no matter how heroic. Thus, if an infected horse were treated very intensively, even with larvicidal anthelmintics, its strongylid egg counts would soon be reduced to zero and would remain there for several weeks. Eventually, however, cyathostomin eggs would reappear in the feces, even if the horse had been housed in sterile conditions. From a control standpoint, this means that horses always transport a source of future cyathostomin populations with them to a new environment. Thus, the so-called "treat and move" strategies that have worked so well for control of ruminant parasites were never quite as successful in horses. In summary, eradication of cyathostomins is neither feasible nor desirable.

Bots (*Gasterophilus* spp.)

The adult stages of stomach bots are flies (dipterans), which share a common seasonality with most other free-living arthropods. Thus, eggs are deposited on the haircoat of the host during late spring through autumn, but fly activity ceases, as legend would have it, with the occurrence of regular frosts in late autumn in temperate areas. Bot instars over-winter within the host as a strategy for avoiding harsh climatic conditions in the environment. Due to seasonality, parasitic bot stages (instars in the oral cavity and alimentary tract) are present during summer and autumn, and acquisition continues until oviposition is terminated.

From a control standpoint, single boticidal treatments are most effective when administered after oviposition by adult stages has ceased, usually in late autumn of each year.

Adaptation to control efforts

Any genetically based adaptation to control efforts should be viewed as an attempt to survive and propagate another generation. Although anthelmintic-resistant nematodes survive treatment to persist as individuals, it is of greater evolutionary significance that their reproductive efficiency remains virtually unimpaired.

Yet other biological adaptations to counteract control attempts could be inferred from certain parasitologic irregularities. For example, both ascarids and pinworms were traditionally considered to be parasites of juvenile horses, so much so that their occurrence in mature animals was worthy of comment in case histories and other published reports. In recent years, however, many practitioners have encountered both patent ascarid infections and problematic pinworm infections in adult horses. One feasible explanation for these atypical observations is that the nematode populations are simply adapting, out of necessity, to a broader array of hosts. In feral horse bands, a significant portion of the entire population is comprised of juveniles year after year. Therefore, access of pinworms and ascarids to a naïve class of host is ensured. In confined herds, however, reproduction is managed and juveniles may disappear entirely from the herd structure on some farms. In managed herds that still include juveniles, the younger horses are often the focus of intensive deworming efforts,

so non-traditional refuges from intensive treatment, such as adult horses, would be advantageous for the parasites in either case.

Shortened egg reappearance periods are discussed in Chapters 8 and 10 in relation to emerging anthelmintic resistance, but they may also represent another example of adaptation to control efforts. It is plausible that anthelmintic treatments applied at regular intervals throughout the year will select for parasite strains that complete their life cycles within a shorter time and start to produce a subsequent generation more rapidly than average. However, this theory has not been substantiated in research studies (Kooyman *et al.*, 2016) and the current evidence suggests that shortened egg reappearance periods are primarily associated with anthelmintic resistance (Chapter 8).

In addition to the positive benefits of parasite control efforts (decreased contamination, lower worm burdens, increased productivity), practitioners must also begin to consider the potential costs in terms of selection pressure and diminished biological diversity. When challenged so intensively, parasites must either adapt or die, and Mother Nature abhors extinction.

References

Chubb, J.C., Ball, M.A., and Parker, G.A. (2009) Living in intermediate hosts: evolutionary adaptations in larval helminths. *Trends Parasitol.*, 26, 93–102.

Duncan, J.L. (1974) Field studies on the epidemiology of mixed strongyle infection in the horse. *Vet. Rec.*, 94, 337–345.

Fabiani, J.V., Lyons, E.T., and Nielsen, M.K. (2016) Dynamics of *Parascaris* and *Strongylus* spp. parasites in untreated juvenile horses. *Vet. Parasitol.*, 30, 62–66.

Gibson, T.E. (1953) The effect of repeated anthelmintic treatment with phenothiazine on fecal egg counts of housed horses, with some observations on the life cycle of *Trichonema* spp. in the horse. *J. Helminthol.*, 27, 29–40.

Herd, R.P. (1986) Epidemiology and control of equine strongylosis at Newmarket. *Equine Vet. J.*, 18, 447–452.

Kooyman, F.N.J., van Doorn, D.C.K., Geurden, T., *et al.* (2016) Species composition of larvae cultured after anthelmintic treatment indicates reduced moxidectin susceptibility of immature *Cylicocyclus* species in horses. *Vet. Parasitol.*, 227, 77–84.

Kuzmina, T.A., Lyons, E.T., Tolliver, S.C., *et al.* (2012) Fecundity of various species of strongylids (Nematoda: Strongylidae) – parasites of domestic horses. *Parasitol. Res.*, 111, 2265–2271.

Poynter, D. (1954) Seasonal fluctuations in the number of strongyle eggs passed in horses. *Vet. Rec.*, 66, 74–78.

Reinemeyer, C.R. and Nielsen, M.K. (2014) Review of the biology and control of *Oxyuris equi*. *Equine Vet. Educ.*, 26, 584–591.

Reinemeyer, C.R., Smith, S.A., Gabel, A.A., and Herd, R.P. (1986) Observations on the population-dynamics of 5 cyathostome nematode species of horses in Northern USA. *Equine Vet. J.*, 18, 121–124.

Sinniah, B. (1982) Daily egg production of *Ascaris lumbricoides*: the distribution of eggs in the faeces and the variability of egg counts. *Parasitology*, 84, 167–175.

Section II

Principles of Equine Parasite Control

6

Decreasing Parasite Transmission by Non-chemical Means

In order to standardize the concepts discussed in the following chapter, let us introduce some relevant technical terms that are not interchangeable.

Definitions

Contamination: the introduction of reproductive products (*e.g.*, strongyle eggs) into the environment. Contamination is initiated by the host and, for most equine parasites, is implemented through defecation.

Translation: a series of events that transforms a reproductive product (*e.g.*, a strongyle egg) into an infective stage (*e.g.*, third stage larva). For most nematode parasites of any importance to equids, translation invariably occurs outside the host in the environment.

Infectivity: the availability of infective stages in the environment. For equine strongyles, for instance, this equates to infective, third stage larvae. Infectivity is a quality of the environment, not the host, and can be described quantitatively, *e.g.*, numbers of third stage larvae per unit of pasture area or weight of forage. Infectivity represents the risk of infection.

Introduction

Parasitism is a progressive and cyclic process, so it is logical that parasite transmission can be confounded, and future generations prevented, by blocking any single event during the course of a life cycle. Most control efforts to date have focused on those portions of the life cycle occurring within the host and have relied almost exclusively on administration of anthelmintics. In order to disrupt transmission effectively, the chemical tools currently at our disposal must be implemented at some point between infection (*i.e.*, ingestion of infective stages) and contamination (*i.e.*, passage of reproductive stages). However, parasite transmission can also be hindered by various non-chemical strategies directed at the host, parasite, environment, or combinations thereof.

Measures to limit contamination

The major objective of most parasite control efforts is to prevent contamination of the environment with reproductive products of the respective parasites. Once eggs enter the environment (termed "contamination"), further development is almost totally under the control of ambient conditions. Passage of feces that contain parasite eggs carries the threat of imminent infection if contemporary environmental conditions are favorable for translation (hatching of eggs and development into infective stages). Conversely, environmental contamination has essentially no parasitologic consequence during seasons when climatic

Handbook of Equine Parasite Control, Second Edition. Martin K. Nielsen and Craig R. Reinemeyer.
© 2018 John Wiley & Sons, Inc. Published 2018 by John Wiley & Sons, Inc.

conditions are not favorable for translation, or if eggs are deposited in an unsuitable habitat. Whenever the climate or habitat do not support translation, fecal contamination is entirely inconsequential from a control standpoint.

Although contamination is the last chronologic step in the life cycle at which traditional control methods can be implemented, this limitation shouldn't discourage us from theorizing about future approaches with the same objective. For example, a birth-control product that sterilized male or female nematodes would provide extremely effective control, even if it did not kill the adult parasites, because it would reduce environmental contamination with fertile eggs.

The following discussions expand on various practical or theoretical ways in which we could decrease contamination.

Ensuring that feces contain few eggs

Dangerous levels of infectivity do not result when horses with relatively low fecal egg counts defecate on pasture. Horses with fecal egg counts lower than 100–200 eggs per gram (EPG) probably have little impact on pasture infectivity as a whole, even when conditions are favorable for translation (see Chapter 8).

Four conditions explain why the feces of a specific horse might contain relatively few strongyle eggs. The first is that the horse is a low contaminator and its minimal egg counts are the manifestation of a permanent genetic trait. Such low egg counts generally persist for that horse's lifetime, even in the absence of anthelmintic treatment. Accordingly, low contaminators may be given access to pastures at virtually any time and season without negative implications for the remainder of the herd.

The second reason for a low fecal egg count is historical exposure to light levels of infectivity. Nematode parasitism is a quantitative phenomenon and large numbers of worms cannot develop unless the

host was previously exposed to high numbers of infective larvae. Horses in this category most often originate within management systems that limit exposure to infectivity (*e.g.*, constant confinement), feature very low stocking densities (*e.g.*, 1 horse per 5 acres), or occur in regional climates that are not conducive to strongylid translation (*e.g.*, the arid southwestern United States).

The third explanation for low fecal egg counts is recent anthelmintic therapy. Treatment with any effective dewormer (by definition >95% FECR) reliably reduces fecal egg counts for a predictable interval post-treatment. That interval is termed the Egg Reappearance Period (ERP; see Chapter 10 for full discussion). For the duration of the predicted ERP, horses treated with the respective anthelmintic will not be sources of significant pasture contamination. However, if the targeted cyathostomins were resistant to the anthelmintic class just administered, fecal egg shedding would either continue unabated or the ERP would be reduced to a shorter duration.

The fourth and final possible reason for a low or negative fecal egg count is that cyathostomin parasite exposure in previous grazing seasons has stimulated partial immunity to the parasites, which is manifested as reduced parasite egg production (Monahan *et al.*, 1997).

Controlling where defecation occurs

In some metropolitan areas, equids pulling public conveyances must be outfitted with "diapers" to collect feces and thereby prevent soiling of public streets. Although capturing feces is impractical for routine equine management, this measure would effectively preclude contamination of the environment and thereby totally block transmission of most parasites.

A more feasible management tool for limiting environmental contamination would be to restrict pasture access for high contaminator horses (see Chapter 8) during seasons when climatic conditions are favorable for translation.

Regular removal of feces

The consequences of environmental contamination can be minimized if horses defecate in sites from which feces can be removed easily. Horse manure can be collected most completely when the pellets are still intact, so the feces of confined horses should be removed frequently enough to prevent mechanical disruption by the stall occupant(s). Feces deposited on pasture should be collected prior to disruption by precipitation, dung beetles, birds or other insectivores, etc. The optimal timing of such fecal removal depends largely on climate and season as temperature and precipitation affect the rate at which strongyle eggs can hatch and develop to the infective third larval stage (see Chapter 3 for details). Manure may be collected less frequently from bedded paddocks or dirt lots. These venues pose minimal risk for strongyle transmission because they contain no vegetation to provide a protective microhabitat for larval persistence, or the vehicle through which most larvae are ingested by horses.

Quarantine practices

Horses arriving on a new farm should be quarantined before being turned out to pasture with other residents. The parasitologic goal of quarantining is to prevent or minimize the introduction of new or genetically unique parasites that differ from the indigenous population. Examples include a highly pathogenic parasite, such as *Strongylus vulgaris,* which is often absent from many well-managed herds. *Strongylus vulgaris* is not known to be resistant to any of the drug classes currently available, so virtually any broad-spectrum treatment will remove adults. One should remember, however, that not all anthelmintics are effective against the migrating larval stages of *S. vulgaris* or *S. edentatus.*

Horse owners should be particularly concerned about the inadvertent introduction of drug-resistant parasites. Strains of cyathostomins or *Parascaris* spp. that are resistant to specific drug classes can be imported via newly arrived horses. To quarantine new arrivals with positive fecal egg counts, a pragmatic approach is to treat them with the most commonly used drug on the farm and then hold them in confinement until a Fecal Egg Count Reduction Test can be completed 14 days post-treatment. If the result is satisfactory (*i.e.,* ≥95% FECR for most of the drugs; see Chapter 10), the horse can be turned out. If not, it should be treated immediately with another anthelmintic with a different mode of action.

This strategy is far less successful against occult, larval (*i.e.,* non-patent) infections because one cannot demonstrate their presence, and there is no immediate way to evaluate the efficacy of an anthelmintic treatment. Readers are referred to other sections in this volume that address larvicidal therapy of ascarids, large strongyles, and encysted cyathostomins (Chapter 7).

On many farms, a traditional quarantine program consists of merely keeping a new horse in its stall for a few days after anthelmintic treatment and then turning it out to pasture. Presumably, the idea is to allow clearance of the eggs of any new strain from the alimentary tract before releasing the horse to a common grazing venue. However, such procedures can be totally inadequate, as illustrated by case scenario number 5 described in a subsequent section of this book.

Pasture hygiene

Pasture hygiene involves removing feces from pastures on a regular basis. If pastures are cleaned thoroughly at intervals shorter than the time it takes for eggs to develop into infective larvae (see Chapter 3), translation can be disrupted before larvae are available to enter the horses. During the warm months of a grazing season, feces need to be collected at intervals shorter than the 7–10 days required for eggs to develop into third stage larvae. During cooler months, the frequency may be decreased. If possible, unscheduled pasture cleaning should be implemented whenever rainfall ≥1 cm is forecast because heavy precipitation mechanically disrupts fecal pellets and spreads eggs and larvae.

Pasture hygiene is time-consuming and labor-intensive. Fecal removal has been accomplished traditionally with a manure fork or broom and shovel. However, several items of equipment, usually manufactured for maintenance of golf courses, are now available for vacuum-cleaning or mechanical removal of feces from the ground. These units are pulled by tractors or ATVs, and can be extremely efficient. Pasture hygiene is more likely to be implemented on smaller farms with limited land available for grazing. The workload is correspondingly greater on large farms, although top-end breeding or training facilities may have the financial resources to implement this measure, regardless. If implemented meticulously, a pasture hygiene program can nearly eliminate the need for anthelmintic treatments. One study evaluated the effects of removing feces twice weekly using pasture vacuum devices and compared it to anthelmintic treatment regimens. Based on quantitative assessments of infectivity, the pasture hygiene approach yielded an 18-fold reduction in larval numbers, compared to an untreated control group, and was four times more efficient than using anthelmintic treatments alone (Herd, 1986a). These same studies determined that mechanical sweeping was a more feasible approach than using a vacuum apparatus (Herd, 1986b).

Whether manure is collected from stalls or pastures, it should be composted properly to minimize any parasitologic risk. As described in Chapter 3, strongyle larvae and eggs cannot survive temperatures in excess of 40 °C (Nielsen *et al.*, 2007). Effective composting can generate temperatures of 70 °C and should effectively kill preparasitic stages within the manure. One study evaluated the effect of windrow composting on the survival of *Parascaris* eggs and found that all eggs were eliminated within just eight days at temperatures ranging between 35 and 55 °C (95–130 °F) (Gould *et al.*, 2013). As a bonus, strongyle eggs were completely eliminated within just a couple of days. However, thorough composting requires frequent turning of the organic material. If left unturned, a compost heap develops temperature gradients in different strata and conditions in the exterior layers may still be favorable for parasite development. Little is known about the thermal tolerance of *Anoplocephala* eggs, but they would likely be killed by the high temperatures resulting from effective composting.

A potential disadvantage of fecal removal is that the pasture ecosystem loses valuable nutrients and supplemental fertilization may be required. However, after thorough composting, manure can be spread onto pastures with no attendant risk of parasite transmission.

Measures to limit infectivity

Stocking density

Stocking density is the single most important management factor affecting parasite transmission. Whenever pastures are overgrazed, no management intervention can be optimally beneficial. Feral, nomadic horses presumably experienced relatively little parasitic disease, but once horses were domesticated and confined within artificial barriers, they could no longer avoid their nematode neighbors.

Proper stocking density is difficult to define because it depends on numerous factors such as soil type, variety and quality of the herbage, local precipitation, size and nutritional requirements of the horses, etc. As a rule of thumb, one horse per 0.5 to 1 ha (1 to 2 acres) of land should not result in overgrazing, but the best way to assess stocking rate is to evaluate the pasture. Under most conditions, forage in the lawns should be no shorter than 5–7 cm (2–3 inches), and the roughs, where horses defecate, should remain ungrazed.

Regulating stocking rates is often difficult to achieve because both herd size and grazing acreage are finite numbers. The latter cannot be increased easily and human nature tends to expand, rather than diminish, herd size over time. Renting extra land or sending horses away for summer grazing are helpful options, if available. A short-term remedy is to supplement the feed of horses on pasture. As long as forage is not the sole source of nutrients, overgrazing can be delayed, if not prevented. Pasture hygiene is the most efficient solution for parasite control on farms where overstocking and overgrazing are a problem.

Harrowing or mowing pastures

Horses are notoriously hard on pastures. Their hard, sharp hooves cut the turf and compact the soil. In addition, equine fecal piles are more prominent than those of any other grazing species, and the tendency of horses to divide pastures into roughs and lawns results in irregular and overgrown areas. Consequently, most horse owners harrow, or "drag", their pastures to break up and distribute fecal piles, and mow down roughs and tall weeds to create a more uniform appearance. These common management practices can have unintended consequences.

Harrowing is widely believed to reduce parasite transmission because intact fecal pellets provide a protective habitat for strongyle eggs and larvae. Breaking up fecal pellets or disseminating fecal piles over a large area exposes free-living stages to unfavorable environmental conditions. However, distributing feces uniformly over an entire pasture confounds the selective grazing behavior of horses described in Chapter 4 and exposes horses to greater levels of infectivity. Similarly, roughs are foci of retained moisture, which is favorable for larval translation. Mowing roughs and tall weeds contributes to the desiccation of pasture herbage and is widely believed to reduce larval survival. However, it should be noted that strongyle L_3s have been shown to be quite resistant to desiccation (Chapter 3), but this mostly applies when L_3s are harbored by intact fecal balls. Thus, fecal disruption is facilitated by mowing, chain harrowing or dragging, with consequent decreased survival of L_3s when ambient conditions are dry.

It is recommended that horses be removed from any pastures that are being dragged or mowed, but the obvious question is, "How long must the pasture be rested?" The recommended rest period varies with geographic location, climate, season, recent weather, types of forage, stocking density, soil types, etc. In temperate climates with warm but not hot summers, such as northern Europe, northern United States, and Canada, temperatures and moisture levels are likely to favor survival of third stage strongyle larvae for months. Therefore, mowing or dragging can only be recommended for pastures that will not be grazed again within the same season. In tropical and subtropical climates, summer temperatures are often too hot to support significant parasite transmission. Subtropical weather conditions are more favorable for parasite transmission during autumn, winter, and spring, when considerations for and against mowing and dragging pastures are similar to those during summers in northern temperate climates. In hot, arid regions, however, third stage larvae can survive for some time within intact fecal pellets, so mechanical disruption during dry periods would reduce larval survival. See Chapter 3 for more details on development and survival of strongyle stages on pasture.

It is interesting to note that studies performed in the 1930s showed that in areas with cold and snowy winters, dragging pastures at the end of the grazing season markedly reduced winter survival of strongyle larvae (Parnell, 1936). Presumably, disrupting fecal pellets rendered larvae more vulnerable to environmental influences.

Pasture rotation

Pasture rotation is performed for various reasons. Rotation may serve as a method for optimizing the use of pastures as a nutrient source. For this strategy, pastures are rested for relatively short intervals, approximately 2 to 4 weeks to allow herbage re-growth before horses are turned back in.

From a parasitologic standpoint, moving horses from one pasture to another might serve to interrupt the strongyle life cycle and effectively reduce parasite transmission. Timing, however, is the most critical issue. Determining when to re-introduce horses to a pasture grazed earlier in the same season depends on climate and weather. In northern temperate climates, it is unlikely that pasture infectivity will diminish significantly within the same grazing season. As a rule of thumb, a northern pasture needs to be rested until the beginning of the subsequent summer before it can be considered relatively parasite-free. In tropical climates, however, significant reductions of larval counts can be observed after just 2 to 4 weeks of rest (Barger *et al.*, 1994).

In temperate areas, horses could be moved during mid-summer to a pasture that had not been grazed previously during the same season. Hay aftermath (a pasture from which a crop of hay has been cut earlier in the season) is ideal for this program, and such pastures are often ready for grazing by early July.

Mixed or alternate grazing

Alternating hosts of different species on the same pasture has been shown to reduce parasite transmission. The key principle is to interchange two animal species that do not share the same parasites; thus, alternating cattle and horses would be superior to alternating cattle and sheep. The potential benefits of this practice include: (1) more efficient use of pasture as a nutrient source, (2) termination of the life cycle when L_3s are ingested by a non-suitable host, and (3) consumption of the herbage in roughs reduces survival of free-living stages.

Co-grazing cattle and sheep with horses have both been investigated. Mixed grazing reduced parasite transmission, but allowing horses and ruminants simultaneous access to a pasture had the disadvantage of increasing the stocking density. Alternate grazing was generally more effective. However, it should be noted that horses share a few parasites with ruminant species. In one study to investigate the effects of co-grazing Shetland ponies and sheep, the prevalence of *Trichostrongylus axei* increased in the ponies, although overall strongylid infection was reduced (Eysker *et al.*, 1983; Eysker, Jansen, and Mirck, 1986). Similarly, horses can be infected by the liver fluke, *Fasciola hepatica*, and this should be considered in areas where fluke infection is endemic in local ruminants (Quigley *et al.*, 2016).

Mixed or alternate grazing is implemented only rarely, however, perhaps because most horse owners do not simultaneously own adequate numbers of ruminants to effect a successful program. Nonetheless, this is practiced on many horse farms in the British Isles, where horses are often co-grazed with cattle, and sheep are turned out to paddocks and pastures after horses have finished grazing them.

Another grazing strategy, termed the dilution principle, has been studied in cattle and sheep. This practice is based on the observation that older, more resilient animals have smaller worm burdens and exhibit lower fecal egg counts than younger, more susceptible individuals. By co-grazing old and young stock, the older hosts ingest infective larvae with little consequence and the younger animals are exposed to progressively lower infectivity (Nansen *et al.*, 1990). Extrapolating this strategy to horses would involve keeping adult horses and juveniles together on the same pasture.

Another grazing strategy, termed the leader/follower approach, has been described for ruminants (Leaver, 1970). In this system, a pasture is grazed first by a group of young, parasite-susceptible animals (leaders). As expected, these non-immune hosts develop high egg counts and cause serious pasture contamination. The young animals are removed from pasture before infectivity reaches hazardous levels, and older, immune hosts (followers) are introduced. The followers ingest far greater numbers of larvae than the leaders, but with less impact on health and productivity. The basic principle behind this strategy is to let both age groups utilize forage efficiently, but the older animals have sufficient acquired immunity to deal with a serious larval challenge. The leader/follower approach has not been evaluated in horses. However, large breeding farms would have the resources to allow weanlings or yearlings to graze a certain pasture first, and then follow them with a group of mature horses. Similarly, perhaps a pasture could first be grazed by horses with high egg counts (juveniles or known high contaminators), and then followed by another cohort of low contaminators. Presumably, the latter group would maintain low egg counts despite intensive larval exposure. The leader/follower approach remains purely speculative for horses, however, and has not been evaluated scientifically.

Pasture renovation

Pasture renovation should be performed on a regular basis to ensure good herbage quality and to prevent the dominance of weeds. Plowing, cultivation, re-seeding, and fertilization of pastures can also have a significant impact on the free-living stages of resident parasite populations. Strongylid larvae, for instance, not only survive being plowed under the soil to a depth of 30 cm, but they can find their way back to the surface. However, so much energy is expended in this process that larval survival is severely compromised and their infectivity may be similarly impacted.

Ascarid eggs do not share the same limitations. Because the infective stage remains within an egg shell, it cannot return to the soil surface when buried by plowing. Therefore, turning the soil may be a very effective control measure for pastures grazed by foals and yearlings. Studies performed with porcine ascarids have demonstrated that eggs buried in the soil remain viable for several years, and are capable of infecting animals when eggs are returned to the surface by subsequent re-plowing (Mejer, 2006). This scenario is similarly feasible for the eggs of *Parascaris* spp.

Measures to limit translation

Control methods that could be implemented after reproductive products leave the host (*i.e.*, by blocking translation or reducing infectivity) remain the Holy

Grail of applied parasite control. Such novel methodologies would constitute highly desirable approaches, particularly if they were sustainable and did not select for genetic adaptations to the management intervention.

Nematode-trapping fungi

Duddingtonia flagrans is a free-living fungus that occurs naturally in herbivore feces. *Duddingtonia* spores survive passage through the gastrointestinal tracts of livestock and grow in feces after it is passed into the environment. This fungus traps and effectively kills strongyle larvae after they hatch in the feces (Larsen, 1999). Although the potential nematocidal activity of *Duddingtonia* has been demonstrated by numerous *in vitro* and *in vivo* studies, its practical utility has been hampered by the requirement to provide fungal spores in the diet on a daily basis. In addition, the potential reduction of larval numbers by nematophagous fungi has ranged from 30 to 90% (Tavela *et al.*, 2011), which may not be sufficient for effective control. Like so many other approaches, *Duddingtonia* offers good experimental promise, but has not yet found utility under standard management conditions.

Fluorescing compounds

Among the various methods that have been investigated for disrupting larval translation, perhaps the most elegant was the inclusion of erythrosin B, a photodynamic xanthene dye, in the daily rations of sheep and grazing beef cattle. When fed to cattle that were infected with trichostrongylid nematodes, erythrosin B was absorbed by adult female worms and passed into their offspring (Healey, Smith, and Smith, 1992). This "tagged" generation left the host as eggs, but when the larvae hatched, they also contained erythrosin B. It was hypothesized that

larvae developing in the environment would be exposed to sunlight and ultraviolet radiation would cause the erythrosin B to effect phototoxicity and ultimately kill the developing larval stages on pasture.

Incorporation of erythrosin B into infective larvae and inducing its lethal effects worked very well in the laboratory, but was less successful in typical livestock management situations (Hawkins, Johnson-Delivorias, and Heitz, 1986). Its utility was hampered by two, basic, biologic factors. First, bovine nematode larvae spend much of their developmental time within the fecal pat, where they are not exposed to sunlight. Second, larvae migrate subsequently into the thatch layer of pasture forage, where there is also relatively little penetration by ultraviolet light. Similar limitations would be expected if administered to horses. Regardless of the difficulties with implementation, this general approach is fascinating.

In the future, perhaps lethal genes that are activated by environmental triggers can be incorporated into certain worm isolates as a means of effective, translational control. However, equine practitioners must recognize that such unique technologies will first be developed to manage potentially lethal nematodes and that the relatively benign parasitisms of horses must wait in line behind the more dramatic problems of small ruminants and cattle.

Conclusion

Although this chapter discussed multiple, non-chemical approaches to decreasing environmental contamination, the only one that is implemented with any frequency is frequent removal and composting of feces. Other measures could be adopted as well, with minor investments of time and equipment. The main thrust is to reduce reliance on chemicals as the sole control element used on many premises.

References

Barger, I.A., Siale, K., Banks, D.J.D., and Le Jambre, L.F. (1994) Rotational grazing for control of gastrointestinal nematodes of goats in a wet tropical environment. *Vet. Parasitol.*, 53, 109–116.

Eysker, M., Jansen, J., and Mirck, M.H. (1986) Control of strongylosis in horses by alternate grazing of horses and sheep and some other aspects of the epidemiology of strongylidae infections. *Vet. Parasitol.*, 19, 103–115.

Eysker, M., Jansen, J., Wemmenhove, R., and Mirck, M.H. (1983) Alternate grazing of horses and sheep as control for gastro-intestinal helminthiasis in horses. *Vet. Parasitol.*, 13, 273–280.

Gould, J.C., Rossano, M.G., Lawrence, L.M., *et al.* (2013) The effects of windrow composting on the viability of *Parascaris equorum* eggs. *Vet. Parasitol.*, 191, 73–80.

Hawkins, J.A., Johnson-Delivorias, M.H., and Heitz, J.R. (1986) Photodynamic-action of erythrosin B as a toxic mechanism for infective larvae of bovine gastrointestinal nematodes. *Vet. Parasitol.*, 21, 265–270.

Healey, M.C., Smith, M.B., and Smith, L.D. (1992) The phototoxic effect of Erythrosin-B on 3rd-stage larvae of gastrointestinal nematodes in sheep. *Vet. Parasitol.*, 43, 249–257.

Herd, R.P. (1986a) Epidemiology and control of equine strongylosis at Newmarket. *Equine Vet. J.*, 18, 447–452.

Herd, R.P. (1986b) Parasite control in horses: Pasture sweeping. *Mod. Vet. Pract.*, 67, 893–984.

Larsen, M. (1999) Biological control of helminths. *Int. J. Parasitol.*, 29, 139–146.

Leaver, J.D. (1970) A comparison of grazing systems for dairy herd replacements. *J. Agric. Sci., Camb.*, 75, 265–272.

Mejer, H. (2006) Transmission, infection dynamics and alternative control of helminths in organic swine. PhD Thesis, Samfundslitteratur Grafik, The Royal Veterinary and Agricultural University, Copenhagen, Denmark.

Monahan, C.M., Chapman, M.R., Taylor, H.W., *et al.* (1997) Foals raised on pasture with or without daily pyrantel tartrate feed additive: Comparison of parasite burdens and host responses following experimental challenge with large and small strongyle larvae. *Vet. Parasitol.*, 73, 277–289.

Nansen, P., Steffan, P., Monrad, J., *et al.* (1990) Effects of separate and mixed grazing on trichostrongylosis in first- and second-season grazing calves. *Vet. Parasitol.*, 36, 265–276.

Nielsen, M.K., Kaplan, R.M., Thamsborg, S.M., *et al.* (2007) Climatic influences on development and survival of free-living stages of equine strongyles: Implications for worm control strategies and managing anthelmintic resistance. *Vet. J.*, 174, 23–32.

Parnell, I.W. (1936) Notes on the survival of the eggs and free-living larvae of sclerostomes on pasture. *Scient. Agric.*, 16, 391–397.

Quigley, A., Sekiya, M., Egan, S., *et al.* (2016) Prevalence of liver fluke infection in Irish horses and assessment of a serological test for diagnosis of equine fasciolosis. *Equine Vet. J.*, 49, 183–188.

Tavela, A.D., Araujo, J.V., Braga, F.R., *et al.* (2011) Biological control of cyathostomin (Nematoda: Cyathostominae) with nematophagous fungus *Monacrosporium thaumasium* in tropical southeastern Brazil. *Vet. Parasitol.*, 175, 92–96.

7

Pharmaceutical Approaches to Parasite Control

Contributing authors: Dave Leathwick and Christian Sauermann

In the not-too-distant past, various natural products and processed derivatives were administered to horses in hopes of achieving parasite control. These "remedies" included black soup, calomel, aniseed, aloes, antimony, licorice, linseed, and quicksilver (reviewed by Lyons, Tolliver, and Drudge, 1999). One imagines that, in many cases, the cure was worse than the disease. The first historical example of an antiparasitic drug with convincing activity against an equine parasite was carbon disulfide, which was effective against bots (Hall, 1917). Oil of chenopodium was also found to be efficacious against strongyles (Hall, Wilson, and Wigdor, 1918), but it allegedly had severe side effects such as anorexia and weight loss (Lyons, Tolliver, and Drudge, 1999). The first modern dewormer launched for equine usage was phenothiazine in the 1940s, which was followed by piperazine in the 1950s (Lyons, Tolliver, and Drudge, 1999).

Equine parasite control was revolutionized in the early 1960s when the benzimidazole drug class was introduced to market. The launch of these inaugural, modern anthelmintic compounds made it feasible, for the first time in history, to disrupt nematode life cycles and prevent parasite transmission. Scientists, veterinarians, and horse owners began to discuss eradication of parasites as if it were a realistic and desirable goal.

Leading equine parasitologists at the time advocated that life cycle features and transmission patterns be considered to make optimal use of these new anthelmintic drugs. They had observed that it took about two months for strongyle eggs to reappear after deworming a horse with thiabendazole, and recommended that subsequent treatments should be timed accordingly (Drudge and Lyons, 1966). This historical recommendation was the first instance in which an egg reappearance period (ERP) was considered as a parameter in equine parasite control. (See Chapter 10 for a detailed definition of ERP and its implications.) A comprehensive control regimen was devised which featured anthelmintic treatments administered at bimonthly intervals all year long. This regimen was later termed the interval-dose program, and it was rapidly adopted at horse establishments world-wide.

The primary parasitic target for the interval-dose program was *Strongylus vulgaris*, which was highly prevalent at the time and widely considered the major parasitic pathogen of horses. The interval program was highly successful in reducing the prevalence of *S. vulgaris* and associated clinical conditions, but its comprehensive efficacy was ultimately compromised by the development of anthelmintic resistance in populations of cyathostomins and later in *Parascaris*

Handbook of Equine Parasite Control, Second Edition. Martin K. Nielsen and Craig R. Reinemeyer.
© 2018 John Wiley & Sons, Inc. Published 2018 by John Wiley & Sons, Inc.

spp. as well. Anthelmintic resistance was first reported in horses in the 1960s, and it is now recognized in all the drug classes currently labeled as nematode parasiticides for horses (Peregrine *et al.*, 2014). Resistance poses a major threat to the sustainability of chemically based control of equine parasites, and consideration of resistance must be a part of all decisions to treat horses with anthelmintics.

This chapter provides a brief discussion of the anthelmintic drug classes currently available for treatment of equine parasites and outlines different principles of parasite control using anthelmintics.

Anthelmintic drug classes

The number of different anthelmintic classes for use in horses is currently very small. In fact, only three drug classes are labeled for efficacy against nematodes, and only two classes for treatment of cestode infections. Relatively recently, the pharmaceutical industry has developed new anthelmintic classes for non-equid animals, but it has been more than 30 years since a nematocidal drug with a new mode of action was introduced for use in horses.

Benzimidazoles

The mode of activity of the benzimidazole drug class is to disrupt energy metabolism at the cellular level. Benzimidazoles (BZs) bind to the protein tubulin and block its polymerization into microtubules. Microtubules are essential structural elements of many cellular organelles and components, such as telomeres and cilia. Many of these structures are critical to energy metabolism, and BZs are the only currently marketed anthelmintic class that has a primary, antimetabolic mode of activity. Nematodes have very limited organs of energy storage, so they must consume nutrients constantly. By blocking energy metabolism, even temporarily, affected worms basically starve to death, and the stages in the intestinal lumen are expelled over a number of days following treatment.

Historically, thiabendazole, cambendazole, fenbendazole, oxfendazole, oxibendazole, mebendazole, and the pro-benzimidazole febantel were all approved for equine use. Of these, only fenbendazole and oxibendazole are still marketed today for horses in the United States.

Fenbendazole (FBZ) was the first broad-spectrum, equine anthelmintic. Among horse dewormers, the term "broad spectrum" is understood to indicate acceptable efficacy against four target parasites: large strongyles, cyathostomins, *Parascaris*, and *Oxyuris*. When administered at an elevated dosage (10 mg/kg) for five consecutive days, FBZ also exhibited high efficacy against migrating ascarid and large strongyle larvae, as well as against encysted cyathostomin larvae (DiPietro, Klei, and Reinemeyer, 1997; Duncan, Bairden, and Abbott, 1998).

Oxibendazole has been found to be effective against *Strongyloides westeri* at 10 mg/kg (Drudge *et al.*, 1981a, 1981b), and one commercial product in North America has a label claim for 15 mg/kg. Fenbendazole also exhibits activity against this parasite (Drudge *et al.*, 1978, 1981a) and some European countries have issued label claims for elevated dosages (50 mg/kg) of this anthelmintic against *Strongyloides*.

Pyrimidines

The pyrimidines (tetrahydropyrimidines) were first introduced in the 1970s and have been used widely ever since. The pyrimidines that are currently available for horses include pyrantel pamoate (international), pyrantel tartrate (North America), pyrantel embonate (Europe), and morantel tartrate, which is labeled for equine use in Australia. Members of this class act as selective acetylcholine agonists and cause rapid, spastic paralysis of nematodes. Paralyzed worms are unable to conduct coordinated feeding activities and would ultimately starve if not expelled by intestinal peristalsis.

Pyrimidines are effective only against luminal stages because there is no parenteral uptake of the drug. Interestingly, pyrimidines are not labeled for efficacy against luminal fourth stage cyathostomin larvae, which have been shown to survive treatment (Reinemeyer, 2003). Generally, pyrantel pamoate (embonate) is available as a suspension or paste product in most of the world, whereas pyrantel tartrate is manufactured in a pelleted formulation and sold as a daily feed additive in North America only. Morantel tartrate is available as both paste and granule formulations in Australia. The pyrimidines are considered to be broad spectrum (large strongyles, cyathostomins, ascarids, pinworms), but also have good efficacy against the tapeworm *Anoplocephala perfoliata*. The label dosage (6.6 mg/kg) typically affords better than 80% cestocidal efficacy (Lyons *et al.*, 1988), but the activity of a double dose (13.2 mg/kg) is greater than 95% (Reinemeyer *et al.*, 2006).

The scientific literature reports no efficacy data for any of the pyrantel salts against *S. westeri*, so it should be assumed that the pyrimidine drug class is ineffective against this parasite. Similarly, some efficacy has been found against *Oxyuris equi* but parasite reductions varied widely among studies, so this drug class should not be the first choice for pinworms (Reinemeyer and Nielsen, 2014).

Macrocyclic lactones

Ivermectin was introduced in the early 1980s and was the first representative of the macrocyclic lactone group. This drug class is very broad and comprises both antibiotics and antiparasitics. Accordingly, the subgroups of macrocyclic lactones with antiparasitic properties are more precisely termed avermectins and milbemycins (Sangster, 1999). For equine use, the avermectin group is represented by ivermectin and abamectin, and the milbemycin group by moxidectin.

Avermectins/milbemycins are known to interfere with the function of glutamate-gated chloride channels, resulting in flaccid paralysis. Paralyzed parasites are unable to ingest nutrients or actively maintain their anatomic location, so those dwelling in the gastrointestinal lumen are expelled by peristalsis. The onset of activity is rapid against intestinal stages, like the pyrimidines, occurring within the first 48 hours post-treatment. Interestingly, avermectin/milbemycin treatment appears to predispose migrating large strongyle stages to being killed by cellular immune responses occurring within a few weeks following treatment (Slocombe *et al.*, 1987). The mechanism behind this phenomenon is not understood.

The avermectins and milbemycins share many properties, but there are a few important exceptions. These drugs are termed endectocides, meaning they kill internal (endo-) as well as external (ecto-) parasites, because both exhibit activity against nematodes and arthropods. In addition to killing all luminal stages of nematodes, ivermectin and moxidectin are very effective against migrating or tissue-dwelling larvae, including those of large strongyles, ascarids, and *Strongyloides*. Efficacy against arthropods includes *Gasterophilus* instars attached to the walls of the stomach and duodenum (Reinemeyer *et al.*, 2000), and ivermectin is labeled for activity against earlier stages residing in the oral cavity. Both drugs have high efficacy against microfilariae of *Onchocerca* spp. in horses (Mancebo, Verdi, and Bulman, 1997; Monahan *et al.*, 1995a). The adult worms residing in deep connective tissues, however, are not killed by macrocyclic lactones, but apparently are rendered infertile for intervals of several months following treatment. Compounds of this class are also effective against larvae of the spirurid nematodes *Habronema* and *Draschia*, which are stomach worms, but can cause granulomatous, cutaneous lesions as well. Neither compound has any efficacy against tapeworms.

Moxidectin was introduced in the mid-1990s and is more lipophilic than ivermectin. Moxidectin accumulates in fatty tissues, which serve as a depot from which the drug is released gradually over time. Consequently, moxidectin differs from ivermectin in two important ways. First, moxidectin demonstrates activity against encysted cyathostomins, with efficacies ranging between 60 and 80% in various studies (Xiao, Herd, and Majewski, 1994; Monahan *et al.*, 1995b, 1996). Accordingly, in North America, moxidectin is labeled for larvicidal efficacy, but only against late third stage and fourth stage encysted cyathostomin larvae (LL_3/L_4). In Europe, however, moxidectin is labeled for activity against both larval categories, and this is supported by recent studies reporting a 60–70% reduction of EL3s following moxidectin administration (Reinemeyer, Prado, and Nielsen, 2015; Bellaw *et al.*, 2018). Second, moxidectin was reported to suppress strongyle egg counts for 16 to 22 weeks post-treatment (Jacobs *et al.*, 1995; DiPietro *et al.*, 1997; Demeulenaere *et al.*, 1997). This was the longest ERP of any anthelmintic approved for horses, and nearly twice that of ivermectin.

Ivermectin (200 µg/kg) has a label claim for *Strongyloides westeri*. Moxidectin (400 µg/kg) was shown to be effective as well (Costa *et al.*, 1998), but readers are reminded that moxidectin use in juveniles may be limited by label restrictions in certain countries.

Piperazine

Piperazine adipate was commonly used to deworm horses several decades ago, but the drug is no longer sold for equine use in most countries. Piperazine works as a gamma-aminobutyric acid (GABA) agonist and evokes spastic paralysis. Piperazine demonstrated good efficacy against *Parascaris* spp. and cyathostomins, but not against large strongyles, pinworms, or bots (Drudge and Lyons, 1986). Historically, piperazine was largely employed as a co-treatment with some benzimidazoles that had little or only modest efficacy against ascarids (*e.g.*, thiabendazole, mebendazole). Arguably, piperazine might demonstrate similar utility today when used with a benzimidazole against BZ-resistant cyathostomins or with a macrocyclic lactone against ML-resistant ascarids. Piperazine's biggest drawbacks are a high dosage (110 mg/kg) and relatively dilute formulations that require voluminous doses administered by nasogastric intubation. In recent years, some veterinarians have revived the practice of administering liquid piperazine formulations to foals via a nasogastric tube, and on some occasions it is combined with other anthelmintics. A recent study investigated the efficacy of piperazine in foals when administered alone or in combination with oxibendazole. Variable but reasonable efficacies were observed against ascarids and strongyles (Lyons, Dorton, and Tolliver, 2016). The study did not observe any clear differences between piperazine when administered alone or in combination with oxibendazole, however. Overall, higher efficacies were observed against ascarids compared to strongyles. These data illustrate that the use of piperazine may still have some merit in foals, but more data are needed to fully evaluate its potential.

Praziquantel

Praziquantel is a member of the quinolone–pyrazine drug group, and its only application in horses is against tape-worms. Praziquantel (PRZ) acts by damaging the tegument of the parasite and by modulating cell membrane permeability, which results in spastic paralysis.

Praziquantel has been used in dogs and cats for decades but was approved for horses only relatively recently. Reported efficacies of PRZ against *Anoplocephala perfoliata* are very high (99 to 100%) (Lyons, Tolliver, and Ennis, 1998).

Other drug classes

During recent years, three new drug classes have been developed for treatment of nematode infections of domestic animals. To date, none of these has been marketed for use in horses. It is largely unknown whether they would be effective against equine parasites, safe for horses, or economically feasible to manufacture for large livestock. A brief account of each new drug class follows.

Emodepside
Emodepside belongs to the cyclooctadepsipeptide class and causes paralysis in nematodes by stimulating latrophilin receptors. Emodepside is approved for use in dogs and cats only, and is primarily effective against hookworms and ascarids.

Derquantel
Derquantel belongs to the spiroindole group and works as an acetylcholine antagonist, causing flaccid paralysis. It is currently marketed in combination with abamectin for use in sheep in New Zealand, Australia, and the United Kingdom, but is likely to be available in other countries in the near future. Derquantel has good efficacy against major trichostrongylid nematodes of sheep. Unfortunately, initial studies have found the drug to be toxic to horses, so it will not be developed as an equine product.

Monepantel
Monepantel is an amino-acetonitrile derivative (AAD) and acts on a specific acetylcholine receptor subunit in nematodes to elicit paralysis. It is broad spectrum, with high efficacy against major gastrointestinal parasites of sheep. It is currently marketed for sheep in Europe, New Zealand, and Australia, but it remains unknown whether this class will be investigated for equine use.

Adverse reactions to anthelmintic therapy

Despite the fact that prevention of clinical disease remains one of the traditional motivations for deworming horses, anthelmintic treatment occasionally triggers specific parasitic problems, even if administered according to label directions. Some of these parasitic syndromes are associated with guarded to poor prognoses, so it is important to recognize these risks and to take appropriate precautions to minimize the threat.

Ascarid impaction of the small intestine

Although ascarid impactions can occur spontaneously, they are most often triggered by prior deworming with an anthelmintic that has a paralytic mode of action (Nielsen, 2016). In a recent review of published impaction cases, 24 of 37 horses had been treated with an anthelmintic prior to the incident. Of these, pyrantel (11) and ivermectin (10) were used most commonly, while benzimidazoles and trichlorfon were documented in one and two incidents, respectively (Nielsen, 2016). Ivermectin, pyrantel salts, and trichlorfon all have paralytic modes of action, which would kill nematodes more rapidly than the metabolic disruption inflicted by BZs. Based on this property, perhaps benzimidazoles should be recommended as a drug of choice for treatment of adult *Parascaris* spp. infections, particularly when large worm burdens are suspected.

Horses with ascarid impactions are usually less than one year of age with a median of five months, but one case in a five-year-old has been reported (Tatz *et al.*, 2012). Of 37 horses undergoing surgery, 31 survived until discharge from the hospital, but only 11 were still alive 12 months later (Nielsen, 2016). The prognosis worsens in complicated cases involving intussusceptions, intestinal rupture, or volvulus.

The timing of ascarid treatments can be a complicated matter. On the one hand, ascarid larvae return to the gut by about four weeks post-infection, and the individual worms continue to increase in size until approximately three months of age. The risk of impaction is likely to increase with the size of the worms. Therefore, an initial anthelmintic treatment at weaning carries a greater risk of adverse sequelae than if the first ascarid treatment had been administered earlier during the suckling phase. In contrast, the efficacy of anthelmintic treatment against any nematode generally improves as the individual worm ages. A case in point, the efficacy of oxibendazole (10 mg/kg) against patent (*i.e.*, mature) ascarid infections ranged from 94% (Lyons *et al.*, 2008) to 100% (Drudge *et al.*, 1979) when measured by FECRT, whereas the same dosage only removed 44.5% of ascarids from the gut when infections were 28 days old (Austin *et al.*, 1991). Considering these conflicting properties, adulticidal ascarid treatments should not begin until foals are at least 60 days of age and should be administered at the maximum tolerable intervals to minimize selection for resistance. In general, the concept of frequently applied, suppressive treatments is no longer recommended for ascarid control. Indeed, some environmental contamination with ascarid eggs may be desirable because

it constitutes environmental refugia (see Chapter 8).

Larval cyathostominosis

Larval cyathostominosis can also occur spontaneously, but more typically it follows an anthelmintic treatment within two weeks prior to the onset of clinical signs (Reid *et al.*, 1995). Horses at risk are typically less than five years old and were treated recently with a non-larvicidal drug during a season when active transmission was minimal. In other words, it tends to happen when a majority of the cyathostomin burden is comprised of encysted larvae. In a cold, temperate climate, most cases of larval cyathostominosis occur during late autumn, winter, and early spring, whereas the onset tends to occur during summer and early autumn in warmer climates. Considering that virtually all horses are infected with cyathostomins, this complication remains an extremely rare event. Horses that develop the syndrome may have a history of management circumstances that allowed them to accumulate large burdens of encysted larvae. Examples include inadequate or ineffective treatments during the preceding grazing season or exposure to over-stocked and highly infective pastures.

Deworming young horses for strongyles during seasons when encysted larvae are most numerous should be performed with care, and one might give serious consideration to larvicidal anthelmintic regimens at that time. Although one of the authors (MKN) has observed larval cyathostominosis following treatment with a larvicidal anthelmintic, the risk appears to be considerably lower. Two choices currently exist for cyathostomin larvicidal therapy: (1) a five-day course of fenbendazole (7.5 or 10 mg/kg) and (2) a single dose of moxidectin (400 µg/kg). Both options historically exhibited good efficacies against encysted burdens, but resistance to the larvicidal fenbendazole regimen has been reported recently (see Chapter 8). In addition, studies have reported a minimal inflammatory reaction in the mucosal membranes after moxidectin treatment (Steinbach *et al.*, 2006; Reinemeyer, 2003), whereas one study found substantial inflammation following fenbendazole use (Steinbach *et al.*, 2006). Three recent studies, however, reported very subtle inflammatory reactions to both moxidectin and fenbendazole treatment (Nielsen *et al.*, 2013; 2015; Steuer *et al.*, submitted). In consideration of these factors, moxidectin should be the drug of choice for horses at risk of developing larval cyathostominosis. Similarly, moxidectin remains the drug of choice for treating a horse with any severe clinical condition caused by cyathostomins.

Post-dosing colics

An effective anthelmintic program clearly reduces the prevalence of colic in a herd over time (Uhlinger, 1990; Hillyer *et al.*, 2002), but an elevated risk of colic has been reported during the initial, post-treatment period (Kaneene *et al.*, 1997; Cohen, Gibbs, and Woods, 1999; Barrett *et al.*, 2005). Such colics could be attributed to mechanical obstruction if ascarids had been present. This would be rare in mature horses, however, and it has been hypothesized that mucosal reactions to the expulsion of dead worms or the release of chemical or immunologic mediators might affect intestinal motility or the alimentary blood supply (Love, 1992).

Anaphylactic reactions

Although it is intuitively feasible that the death of parasites within tissues could result in anaphylaxis, the treatment of migrating strongyles, ascarids, and encysted cyathostomins has not been associated with adverse events of this type. In fact, studies evaluating the effects of ivermectin and moxidectin have found good healing of parasitic lesions with only limited inflammatory reaction to the dead nematodes (Slocombe *et al.*, 1987; Reinemeyer, 2003; Steinbach *et al.*, 2006; Nielsen *et al.*, 2015). The rare examples of anaphylactic reactions following anthelmintic treatment have been associated with treatment of filarial parasites, particularly *Onchocerca* spp. (Mancebo, Verdi, and Bulman, 1997; Wildenburg *et al.*, 1994) and *Dirofilaria immitis* infection in dogs (Boreham and Atwell, 1983). Horses harboring *Onchocerca* spp. infection may experience milder inflammatory reactions following treatment with moxidectin compared to ivermectin (Mancebo, Verdi, and Bulman, 1997; Monahan *et al.*, 1995a).

Anthelmintic toxicosis

Although this happens very rarely, some cases of anthelmintic toxicosis have been described in the literature. These are most commonly reported for the avermectin/milbemycins, which are very lipophilic drugs that can sometimes cross the blood/brain barrier.

Ivermectin toxicosis has been described in foals as well as adult horses (Swor, Whittenburg, and Chaffin, 2009; Bruenisholz *et al.*, 2012). Symptoms occur about 18-24 hours post treatment and include depression, ataxia, lip drooping, muscle fasciculation, and bilateral mydriasis (Swor *et al.*, 2009). Treatment options include charcoal administered via nasogastric tube, anti-inflammatory medication, fluid therapy and lipid emulsion (Bruenisholz *et al.*, 2012). One study suggested that ivermectin toxicosis could occur in horses that were administered correct doses of ivermectin but simultaneously were exposed to toxic *Solanum*-type plants in the hay (Norman *et al.*, 2012). Similarly, moxidectin toxicosis has been reported in foals given between 2.5 and 12.8 times the approved label dosage (Khan, Kuster, and Hansen, 2002). Clinical signs are similar to those described for ivermectin toxicosis, but tend to be more pronounced and foals can present in a completely flaccid, paralyzed state. Affected foals can recover if provided appropriate supportive therapy, but the prognosis is guarded if the condition is pronounced. Again, readers are reminded that moxidectin is not labeled for administration to foals in most countries.

Anthelmintic treatment regimens

A variety of treatment programs have been described over the years, but most were based on the principles of the interval-dose program, which was introduced in the 1960s (Drudge and Lyons, 1966). Essentially, these treatment regimens attempted to prevent or reduce parasite transmission, but often without adequate consideration of the size or the composition of the parasite burden. With the advent of efficacious, broad-spectrum dewormers in the 1960s, the achievement and perpetual maintenance of parasite-free premises was considered a realistic goal. The cumulative experiences of intervening decades, however, have demonstrated that the parasite-free horse farm does not exist, and attempts to impose such a venue on Mother Nature merely create strong selective pressure for the development of anthelmintic resistance. Modern parasite control strategies, therefore, have evolved toward acceptance of some level of parasitism and maintenance of sustainable control objectives. The following section offers a brief description of the main therapeutic approaches that have been applied historically to achieve equine parasite control (Love, 1993).

Interval-dose program

As mentioned previously, interval dosing involves treatment of all horses on a farm at fixed intervals, all year long. The original, recommended treatment interval was two months, but timing should be adjusted to match the expected egg reappearance period (ERP) of the anthelmintic used. Interval dosing is an example of suppressive treatment, in which the objective is to minimize contamination by matching treatment intervals with the ERPs of effective products.

Historically, interval-dose programs have not involved parasite surveillance, diagnostics, or evaluation of anthelmintic efficacy. Furthermore, climatic influences and seasonal differences in parasite transmission were given little, if any, consideration. Rather, rote utilization of broad-spectrum anthelmintics at prescribed intervals was considered the only strategy necessary to ensure control of all important parasites.

The principles of the interval-dose program are very simple and easy to implement. It is a one-size-fits-all, cook-book recipe that does not require expenditures for diagnostic surveillance or consideration of complicating factors such as age of horses, stocking densities, or seasonal variations. As a result, interval-dosing has become the universal standard in managed horse populations world-wide (Lloyd et al., 2000; O'Meara and Mulcahy, 2002; Robert et al., 2015). However, most equine parasitologists now believe that the interval-dose program and its derivatives have been the major factors responsible for the current high levels of anthelmintic resistance at equine establishments (Kaplan and Nielsen, 2010), and this approach is almost certainly not sustainable in the long term.

Strategic dosing

As opposed to interval dosing, strategic dosing takes seasonal differences into consideration. In this program, treatments are primarily administered during the active grazing season, but are usually still performed without diagnostic information. Hence, all horses receive the same treatments at fixed times during the year, and the treatment intensity can be lowered considerably in comparison to the interval-dose approach.

Continuous, daily treatment

This approach involves the daily administration of pyrantel tartrate to selected horses, either perennially or just throughout the grazing season. Daily administration of pyrantel tartrate should kill ingested L_3s before they invade mucosal tissues, and would have additional therapeutic activity against recently emerged adults. Consequently, egg counts of horses receiving daily pyrantel tartrate should remain low while receiving the regimen. Due to national differences in drug approvals and marketing strategies, daily pyrantel tartrate formulations are only available in North America. Recent investigations have documented that while egg counts can be significantly lowered in horses kept on a daily pyrantel tartrate regimen, strongyle egg counts are not reduced to 0, and seasonal (Reinemeyer *et al.*, 2014) or gradual (Bellaw *et al.*, 2016) increases can be observed regardless.

Selective therapy

Selective therapy (or targeted treatment) is markedly different from the control strategies described previously because it abandons whole-herd treatment and designates only certain individual horses for anthelmintic therapy. Selective therapy reduces treatment intensity and selection for resistance by considering the distribution of parasites in mature members of the herd. In technical terms, selective therapy creates horse *refugia* by leaving a proportion of the parasite population untreated (see Chapter 3 for a definition of *parasite refugia*).

As a general rule, parasites are always over-dispersed among their hosts (Galvani, 2003) so that a minority of animals harbors a majority of the parasites. It is entirely logical to allocate specific treatments to these "wormy" individuals, while others in the herd are dewormed less frequently, and possibly even left untreated. Implementation of this approach requires systematic surveillance with tools that are capable of categorizing infection intensity. A number of diagnostic methods have been employed to identify and segregate hosts with differing susceptibilities to parasitism. In ruminants, for example, this principle has been implemented by classifying gradations of mucosal pallor as an indication of anemia caused by the highly pathogenic trichostrongylid, *Haemonchus contortus*. This system, known as FAMACHA® (Malan, van Wyk, and Wessels, 2001), has proven highly useful for small ruminants in areas where *Haemonchus contortus* predominates. Other proposed methods of selecting individuals for treatment are based on body-condition scoring or regular body weights, and treating only those with weight loss or suboptimal weight gain (reviewed by van Wyk *et al.*, 2006).

Recommendations for selective therapy of horses are based on quantitative fecal analysis of all mature equids on the premises, and treatment of only those with counts exceeding a predetermined cut-off value (Gomez and Georgi, 1991; Duncan and Love, 1991). The selection of threshold values for treatment has been a contentious issue because one standard value might not be equally valid for different parasites, horses, geographies, or management systems. Until recently, the choice of cut-off values has not been evidence-based because no equine studies had investigated the relationship between egg counts and worm counts. One paper compared the designated cut-off

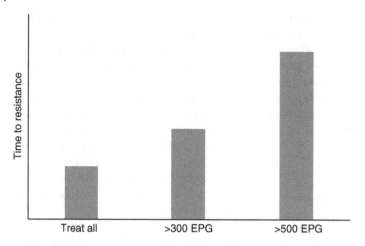

Figure 7.1 Simulation of three different anthelmintic treatment regimens applied to adult horses in Kentucky, USA. In the "treat all" regimen, all horses received ivermectin three times per year in April, August, and November. The other two regimens represent selective treatments that were administered only to horses whose strongyle egg counts exceeded two different cut-off values: 300 or 500 eggs per gram (EPG). Fecal egg counts were assessed at the same three time points for all groups. The *y*-axis represents the time required for resistance to develop with each treatment regimen.

values used by a number of parasitology laboratories and found a weak consensus for anthelmintic treatment when egg counts reached approximately 200 EPG (Uhlinger, 1993). Based on historical egg count and worm count data generated over 50 years of research at the University of Kentucky, it was recently reported that no direct, linear relationship could be established between egg counts and worm burdens. However, it was determined that horses with strongylid egg counts between 100 and 500 EPG harbored significantly smaller worm burdens than those with egg counts exceeding this EPG range (Nielsen *et al.*, 2010). These findings support the establishment of a threshold value in the 100 to 500 EPG range. However, a large majority of the horses in the Kentucky data set were less than two years of age, and selective therapy is currently being promoted only for mature horses.

Evaluation of a data set of fecal egg counts from horse herds in the southeastern United States revealed that only one-half of the horses represented would have

been treated if a hypothetical cut-off value of 200 EPG had been implemented (Kaplan *et al.*, 2004). Still, using a drug with 99% efficacy in those populations would have reduced the strongyle egg contamination from the overall herd by 96% (Kaplan and Nielsen, 2010).

A computer simulation model for the entire cyathostomin life cycle has recently been developed. This model imports weather station data from a given region and can be used to test different treatment scenarios and their impact on the development of anthelmintic resistance over time. Figure 7.1 presents a model output from one such simulation. Ten years of climatic data from a weather station in Central Kentucky, USA were imported into the model and a herd of horses was simulated over 40 model years. In the simulated scenario, three treatment strategies were applied. In one scenario, all horses were treated three times a year (April, August, and November) with ivermectin, while in the other two a selective treatment approach was applied with treatment thresholds of 300 or 500 EPG. The graphic data demonstrate that the two selective treatment regimens considerably delayed the development of resistance.

Concerns have been raised regarding the risk of clinical disease when implementing selective therapy in horses (Nielsen, Pfister, and von Samson-Himmelstjerna, 2014). The consequences of under-treatment have not yet been evaluated, but we are reminded that cyathostomins are generally not very pathogenic and clinical disease is the rare exception rather than the rule. Consider that the most efficient strategy for avoiding further development of anthelmintic resistance in equine parasites is to simply stop deworming horses. However, as pointed out earlier in this chapter, it is a universal goal to prevent parasitic disease, so some anthelmintic treatments will be needed in the large majority of cases. Complexity arises when we try to strike that subtle balance between treating too little and treating too much.

In several European countries, anthelmintic use is legally restricted to therapeutic applications, and rote or preventive treatments are not permitted. As a result, selective therapy is used widely for Danish and Swedish horses, and recent studies have determined that *Strongylus vulgaris* is exhibiting resurgence in prevalence on many farms, mostly in asymptomatic horses (Bracken *et al.*, 2012; Nielsen *et al.*, 2012; Werell, 2017). The strict disallowance of prophylactic treatments has resulted in a significant share of horses not receiving any treatments if they consistently have low egg counts. This extreme example illustrates how a parasite control program should not be based solely on regular fecal egg counts to support the selective therapy principle. A holistic approach, therefore, combines parasite surveillance to monitor contamination levels, rigorous evaluation of anthelmintic efficacy, and strategic treatments specifically to maintain control over non-cyathostomin parasites, such as large strongyles and tapeworms. These philosophies are reflected in the current parasite control guidelines published by the American Association for Equine Practitioners (Nielsen *et al.*, 2016).

Combination deworming

The ever-increasing levels of anthelmintic resistance and the absence of new drug classes for the equine market have forced the industry to consider alternative uses of the existing portfolio of anthelmintic products. One example is the use of so-called combination deworming, whereby two or more anthelmintics that target the same parasites are incorporated into a single, simultaneous treatment. It should be emphasized that this differs from the use of existing anthelmintic combinations (*e.g.*, ivermectin plus praziquantel) that target different types of parasites, such as nematodes and cestodes. Several combination products (*i.e.*, two drugs with overlapping nematocidal spectra) are already marketed in New Zealand and Australia (Scott, Bishop, and Pomroy, 2015; Wilkes *et al.*, 2017), and some veterinary practitioners elsewhere are employing combination strategies on an extra-label basis (Lyons, Dorton, and Tolliver, 2016).

The concept of combination deworming is supported by a growing body of scientific evidence in small ruminants, where it has been shown to be more sustainable than rotating between the same active ingredients (Leathwick *et al.*, 2012; Bartram *et al.*, 2012). The aforementioned cyathostomin model has made similar predictions for the value of combination therapy in horses. Figure 7.2 presents output from one such simulation, wherein horses were treated six times a year, which is common practice for some horse farms (Robert *et al.*, 2015). The simulation compared treating all horses with the same anthelmintic (ivermectin) throughout the year to rotation between the three available anthelmintic

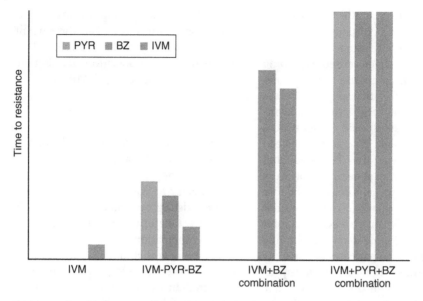

Figure 7.2 Simulation outputs predicting how quickly resistance would develop to four different anthelmintic treatment regimens applied to adult horses in Kentucky, USA. In each simulated scenario, all horses were treated at six, regularly spaced intervals per year. In the "IVM" scenario, all horses received ivermectin at every treatment. In the "IVM-PYR-BZ" scenario, treatments were rotated among three drug classes: ivermectin, pyrantel, and a benzimidazole. In the two combination treatment scenarios, the anthelmintic treatments listed were administered simultaneously to all horses. One scenario was a two-way combination featuring ivermectin and a benzimidazole (IVM + BZ) and the other was a three-way combination featuring three drug classes (IVM + PYR + BZ). The y-axis represents the time required for resistance to develop with each treatment regimen.

drug classes and the use of two different potential combinations. It is clear from the graph that combination therapy offered marked advantages over the course of the simulation, with resistance being considerably slower to develop. These results agree strongly with the research conducted in small ruminants. However, one should remember that these are model predictions and must still be verified by field studies.

A recent field study evaluated the efficacy of a combination of pyrantel pamoate and oxibendazole, and found an additive effect of the two anthelmintics when administered in combination (Kaplan *et al.*, 2014). While this was a promising finding, it did not provide any information about the sustainability of this approach over time. More recently, the efficacy of a pyrantel pamoate/oxibendazole combination was followed over

the course of one year in a population of horses harboring cyathostomins known to be resistant to both drug classes. Although an additive effect was observed for the first combination treatment, the efficacy was dramatically reduced thereafter for all subsequent treatments (Scare *et al.*, 2018). It was suggested that the reason for this development was that the combination efficacy did not exceed 80%, which meant that a large proportion of parasites survived the initial, combination treatment and allowed a strong selection for multidrug resistance. The take-home message from this study is that while combination deworming may offer some benefits, it is very important to evaluate the efficacy of each active ingredient against the target parasite population before attempting this approach. Furthermore, ruminant studies strongly suggest the importance of leaving a proportion of animals untreated when utilizing combination deworming to help maintain adequate parasite *refugia* (Leathwick *et al.*, 2012).

References

Austin, S.M., DiPietro, J.A., Foreman, J.H., *et al.* (1991) Comparison of the efficacy of ivermectin, oxibendazole, and pyrantel pamoate against 28-day *Parascaris equorum* larvae in the intestine of pony foals. *J. Am. Vet. Med. Assoc.*, 198, 1946–1949.

Barrett, E.J., Blair, C.W., Farlam, J., and Proudman, C.J. (2005) Postdosing colic and diarrhoea in horses with serological evidence of tapeworm infection. *Vet. Rec.*, 156, 252–253.

Bartram, D.J., Leathwick, D.M., Taylor, M.A., *et al.* (2012) The role of combination anthelmintic formulations in the sustainable control of sheep nematodes. *Vet. Parasitol.*, 186, 151–158.

Bellaw, J.L., Pagan, J., Cadell, S., *et al.* (2016) Objective evaluation of two deworming regimens in young Thoroughbreds using parasitological and performance parameters. *Vet. Parasitol.*, 221, 69–75.

Bellaw J.L., Krebs, K., Reinemeyer, C.R., *et al.* (2018) Anthelmintic therapy of equine cyathostomin nematodes – larvicidal efficacy, egg reappearance period, and drug resistance. *Int. J. Parasitol.*, 48, 97–105.

Boreham, P.F.L. and Atwell, R.B. (1983) Adverse drug reactions in the treatment of filarial parasites: haematological, biochemical, immunological and pharmacological changes in *Dirofilaria immitis* infected dogs treated with diethylcarbamazine. *Int. J. Parasitol.*, 13, 547–556.

Bracken, M.K., Wøhlk, C.B.M., Petersen, S.L., and Nielsen, M.K. (2012) Evaluation of conventional PCR for detection of *Strongylus vulgaris* on horse farms. *Vet. Parasitol.*, 184, 387–391.

Bruenisholz, H., Kupper, J., Muentener, C.R., *et al.* (2012) Treatment of ivermectin overdose in a miniature Shetland pony using intravenous administration of a lipid emulsion. *J. Vet. Intern. Med.*, 26, 407–411.

Cohen, N.D., Gibbs, P.G., and Woods, A.M. (1999) Dietary and other management factors associated with colic in horses. *J. Am. Vet. Med. Assoc.*, 215, 53–60.

Costa, A.J., Barbosa, O.F., Moraes, F.R., *et al.* (1998) Comparative efficacy evaluation of moxidectin gel and ivermectin paste against internal parasites of equines in Brazil. *Vet. Parasitol.*, 80, 29–36.

Demeulenaere, D., Vercruysse, J., Dorny, P., and Claerebout, E. (1997) Comparative studies of ivermectin and moxidectin in the control of naturally acquired cyathostome infections in horses. *Vet. Rec.*, 15, 383–386.

DiPietro, J.A., Klei, T.R., and Reinemeyer, C.R. (1997) Efficacy of fenbendazole against encysted small strongyle larvae. *Proceedings American Association of Equine Practitioners Convention*, 43, 343–344.

DiPietro, J.A., Hutchens, D.E., Lock, T.F., *et al.* (1997) Clinical trial of moxidectin oral gel in horses. *Vet. Parasitol.*, 72, 167–177.

Drudge, J.H. and Lyons, E.T. (1966) Control of internal parasites of horses. *J. Am. Vet. Med. Assoc.*, 148, 378–383.

Drudge, J.H. and Lyons, E.T. (1986) *Internal parasites of equids with emphasis on treatment and control.* Hoechst-Roussel Agri-Vet Company, Somerville, NJ, USA.

Drudge, J.H., Lyons, E.T., and Tolliver, S.C. (1978) Critical and controlled tests and clinical-trials with suspension and granule formulations of anthelmintic, fenbendazole, in horse. *J. Equine Med. Surg.*, 2, 22–26.

Drudge, J.H., Lyons, E.T., Tolliver, S.C., and Kubis, J.E. (1979) Critical tests and clinical trials on oxibendazole in horses with special reference to removal of *Parascaris equorum*. *Am. J. Vet. Res.*, 40, 758–761.

Drudge, J.H., Lyons, E.T., Tolliver, S.C., and Kubis, J.E. (1981a) Clinical-trials with fenbendazole and oxibendazole for *Strongyloides westeri* infection in foals. *Am. J. Vet. Res.*, 42, 526–527.

Drudge, J.H., Lyons, E.T., Tolliver, S.C., and Kubis, J.E. (1981b) Clinical-trials of oxibendazole for control of equine internal parasites. *Mod. Vet. Pract.*, 62, 679–682.

Duncan, J.L. and Love, S. (1991) Preliminary observations on an alternative strategy for the control of horse strongyles. *Equine Vet. J.*, 23, 226–228.

Duncan, J.L., Bairden, K., and Abbott, E.M. (1998) Elimination of mucosal cyathostome larvae by five daily treatments with fenbendazole. *Vet. Rec.*, 142, 268–271.

Galvani, A.P. (2003) Immunity, antigenic heterogeneity, and aggregation of helminth parasites. *J. Parasitol.*, 89, 232–241.

Gomez, H.H. and Georgi, J.R. (1991) Equine helminth infections: control by selective chemotherapy. *Equine Vet. J.*, 23, 198–200.

Hall, M.C. (1917) Notes in regard to bots, *Gastrophilus* spp. *J. Am. Vet. Med. Assoc.*, 52, 177–184.

Hall, M.C., Wilson, R.H., and Wigdor, M. (1918) The anthelmintic treatment of equine intestinal strongylidosis. *J. Am. Vet. Med. Assoc.*, 54, 47–55.

Hillyer, M.H., Taylor, F.G.R., Proudman, C.J., *et al.* (2002) Case control study to identify risk factors for simple colonic obstruction and distension colic in horses. *Equine Vet. J.*, 34, 455–463.

Jacobs, D.E., Hutchinson, M.J., Parker, L., and Gibbons, L.M. (1995) Equine cyathostome infection: suppression of faecal egg output with moxidectin. *Vet. Rec.*, 137, 545.

Kaneene, J.B., Miller, R., Ross, W.A., *et al.* (1997) Risk factors for colic in the Michigan (USA) equine population. *Prev. Vet. Med.*, 30, 23–36.

Kaplan, R.M. and Nielsen, M.K. (2010) An evidence-based approach to equine parasite control: It ain't the 60s anymore. *Equine Vet. Educ.*, 22, 306–316.

Kaplan, R.M., Klei, T.R., Lyons, E.T., *et al.* (2004) Prevalence of anthelmintic resistant cyathostomes on horse farms. *J. Am. Vet. Med. Assoc.*, 225, 903–910.

Kaplan, R.M., West, E.M., Norat-Collazo, L.M., and Vargas, J. (2014) A combination treatment strategy using pyrantel pamoate and oxibendazole demonstrates additive effects for controlling equine cyathostomins. *Equine Vet. Educ.*, 485–491.

Khan, S.A., Kuster, D.A., and Hansen, S.R. (2002) A review of moxidectin overdose cases in equines from 1998 through 2000. *Vet. Human Toxicol.*, 44, 232–235.

Leathwick, D.M., Waghorn, T.S., Miller, C.M., *et al.* (2012) Managing anthelmintic resistance – Use of a combination anthelmintic and leaving some lambs untreated to slow the development of resistance to ivermectin. *Vet. Parasitol.*, 285–294.

Lloyd, S., Smith, J., Connan, R.M., *et al.* (2000) Parasite control methods used by horse owners: factors predisposing to the development of anthelmintic resistance in nematodes. *Vet. Rec.*, 146, 487–492.

Love, S. (1992) The role of equine strongyles in the pathogenesis of colic and current options for prophylaxis. *Equine Vet. J. Suppl.*, 13, 5–9.

Love, S. (1993) Treatment and prevention of intestinal parasite-associated disease. *Vet. Clin. Equine*, 19, 791–806.

Lyons, E.T., Dorton, A.R., and Tolliver, S.C. (2016) Evaluation of activity of fenbendazole, oxibendazole, piperazine, and pyrantel pamoate alone and combinations against ascarids, strongyles, and strongyloides in horse foals in field tests on two farms in Central Kentucky in 2014 and 2015. *Vet. Parasitol. Reg. Stud. Rep.* 3–4, 23–26.

Lyons, E.T., Tolliver, S.C., and Drudge, J.H. (1999) Historical perspective of cyathostomes: prevalence, treatment and control programs. *Vet. Parasitol.*, 85, 97–112.

Lyons, E.T., Tolliver, S.C., and Ennis, L.E. (1998) Efficacy of praziquantel (0.25 mg kg(-1)) on the cecal tapeworm (*Anoplocephala perfoliata*) in horses. *Vet. Parasitol.*, 78, 287–289.

Lyons, E.T., Drudge, J.H., Tolliver, S.C., *et al.* (1988) Determination of the efficacy of pyrantel pamoate at the therapeutic dose against the tapeworm *Anoplocephala perfoliata* in equids using a modification of the critical test. *Vet. Parasitol.*, 31, 13–18.

Lyons, E.T., Tolliver, S.C., Ionita, M., and Collins, S.S. (2008) Evaluation of parasiticidal activity of fenbendazole, ivermectin, oxibendazole, and pyrantel pamoate in horse foals with emphasis on ascarids (*Parascaris equorum*) in field studies on five farms in Central Kentucky in 2007. *Parasitol. Res.*, 103, 287–291.

Malan, F.S., van Wyk, J.A., and Wessels, C.D. (2001) Clinical evaluation of anaemia in sheep: early trials. *Onderstepoort J. Vet. Res.*, 61, 165–174.

Mancebo, O.A., Verdi, J.H., and Bulman, G.M. (1997) Comparative efficacy of moxidectin 2% equine oral gel and ivermectin 2% equine oral paste against *Onchocerca cervicalis* (Railliet and Henry, 1910) microfilariae in horses with naturally acquired infections in Formosa (Argentina). *Vet. Parasitol.*, 73, 243–248.

Monahan, C.M., Chapman, M.R., French, D.D., Klei, T.R. (1995a) Efficacy of moxidectin oral gel against *Onchocerca cervicalis* microfilariae. *J. Parasitol.*, 81, 117–118.

Monahan, C.M., Chapman, M.R., French, D.D., *et al.* (1995b) Dose titration of moxidectin oral gel against gastrointestinal parasites of ponies. *Vet. Parasitol.*, 59, 241–248.

Monahan, C.M., Chapman, M.R., Taylor, H.W., *et al.* (1996) Comparison of moxidectin oral gel and ivermectin oral paste against a spectrum of internal parasites of ponies with special attention to encysted cyathostome larvae. *Vet. Parasitol.*, 63, 225–235.

Nielsen, M.K. (2016) Evidence-based considerations for control of *Parascaris* spp. infections in horses. *Equine Vet. Educ.*, 28, 224–231.

Nielsen, M.K., Pfister, K., and von Samson-Himmelstjerna, G. (2014) Selective therapy in equine parasite control – application and limitations. *Vet. Parasitol.*, 202, 95–103.

Nielsen, M.K., Baptiste, K.E., Tolliver, S.C., *et al.* (2010) Analysis of multiyear studies in horses in Kentucky to ascertain whether counts of eggs and larvae per gram of feces are reliable indicators of numbers of strongyles and ascarids present. *Vet. Parasitol.*, 174, 77–84.

Nielsen, M.K., Vidyashankar, A.N., Olsen, S.N., *et al.* (2012) *Strongylus vulgaris* associated with usage of selective therapy on Danish horse farms – is it reemerging? *Vet. Parasitol.*, 189, 260–266.

Nielsen, M.K., Betancourt, A., Lyons, E.T., *et al.* (2013) Characterization of the inflammatory response to anthelmintic treatment in ponies naturally infected with cyathostomin parasites. *Vet. J.*, 198, 457–462.

Nielsen, M.K., Loynachan, A.T., Jacobsen, S., *et al.* (2015) Local and systemic inflammatory and immunologic reactions to cyathostomin larvicidal therapy in horses. *Vet. Imm. Immunopathol.*, 168, 203–210.

Nielsen, M.K., Mittel, L., Grice, A., *et al.* (2016) *AAEP Parasite Control Guidelines*, American Association of Equine Practitioners, Lexington. www.aaep.org.

Norman, T.E., Chaffin, M.K., Norton, P.L., *et al.* (2012) Concurrent Ivermectin and

Solanum spp. toxicosis in a herd of horses. *J. Vet. Intern. Med.*, 26, 1439–1442.

O'Meara, B. and Mulcahy, G. (2002) A survey of helminth control practices in equine establishments in Ireland. *Vet. Parasitol.*, 109, 101–110.

Peregrine, A.S., Molento, M.B., Kaplan, R.M., and Nielsen, M.K. (2014) Anthelmintic resistance in important parasites of horses: does it really matter? *Vet. Parasitol.*, 201, 1–8.

Reid, S.W., Mair, T.S., Hillyer, M.H., and Love, S. (1995) Epidemiological risk factors associated with a diagnosis of clinical cyathostomiasis in the horse. *Equine Vet. J.*, 27, 127–130.

Reinemeyer, C.R. (2003) Indications and benefits of moxidectin use in horses. *Proceedings, World Equine Veterinary Association*, Buenos Aires, Argentina, 15–17 October, pp. 3–12.

Reinemeyer, C.R. and Nielsen, M.K. (2014) Review of the biology and control of *Oxyuris equi. Equine Vet. Educ.*, 26, 584–591.

Reinemeyer, C.R., Prado, J.C., and Nielsen, M.K. (2015) Comparison of the larvicidal efficacies of moxidectin or a five-day regimen of fenbendazole in horses harbouring cyathostomin populations resistant to the adulticidal dosage of fenbendazole. *Vet. Parasitol.*, 214, 100–107.

Reinemeyer, C.R., Scholl, P.J., Andrews, F.M., and Rock, D.W. (2000) Efficacy of moxidectin equine oral gel against endoscopically-confirmed *Gasterophilus nasalis* and *Gasterophilus intestinalis* (Diptera: *Oestridae*) infections in horses. *Vet. Parasitol.*, 88, 287–291.

Reinemeyer, C.R., Hutchens, D.E., Eckblad, W.P., *et al.* (2006) Dose confirmation studies of the cestocidal activity of pyrantel pamoate paste in horses. *Vet. Parasitol.*, 138, 234–239.

Reinemeyer, C.R., Prado, J.C., Andersen, U.V., *et al.* (2014) Effects of daily pyrantel tartrate on strongylid population dynamics and performance parameters of young horses repeatedly infected with cyathostomins and *Strongylus vulgaris. Vet. Parasitol.*, 204, 229–237.

Robert, M., Hu, W., Nielsen, M.K., and Stowe, C.J. (2015) Attitudes towards implementation of surveillance-based parasite control on Kentucky Thoroughbred farms – current strategies, awareness, and willingness-to-pay. *Equine Vet. J.*, 47, 694–700.

Sangster, N.C. (1999) Pharmacology of anthelmintic resistance in cyathostomes: will it occur with the avermectin/ milbemycins? *Vet. Parasitol.*, 85, 189–204.

Scare, J.A., Lyons, E.T., Wielgus, K.M., *et al.* (2018) Combination deworming for the control of double-resistant cyathostomin parasites – short and long term consequences. *Vet. Parasitol.*, 251, 112–118.

Scott, I., Bishop, R.M., and Pomroy, W.E. (2015) Anthelmintic resistance in equine helminth parasites – a growing issue for horse owners and veterinarians in New Zealand? *N. Z. Vet. J.*, 63, 188–198.

Slocombe, J.O.D., Mccraw, B.M., Pennock, P.W., *et al.* (1987) *Strongylus vulgaris* in the tunica media of arteries of ponies and treatment with ivermectin. *Can. J. Vet. Res.*, 51, 232–235.

Steinbach, T., Bauer, C., Sasse, H., *et al.* (2006) Small strongyle infection: Consequences of larvicidal treatment of horses with fenbendazole and moxidectin. *Vet. Parasitol.*, 139, 115–131.

Steuer, A., Loynachan, A.T., and Nielsen, M.K. (submitted) Evaluation of the mucosal inflammatory responses to larvicidal treatment of equine cyathostomins.

Swor, T.M., Whittenburg, J.L., and Chaffin, K. (2009) Ivermectin toxicosis in three adult horses. *J. Am. Vet. Med. Assoc.*, 235, 558–562.

Tatz, A.J., Segev, G., Steinman, A., *et al.* (2012) Surgical treatment for acute small intestinal obstruction caused by *Parascaris equorum* infection in 15 horses (2002–2011). *Equine Vet. J.*, 44, 111–114.

Uhlinger, C. (1990) Effects of three anthel-mintic schedules on the incidence of colic in horses. *Equine Vet. J.*, 22, 251–254.

Uhlinger, C. (1993) Uses of fecal egg count data in equine practice. *Comp. Cont. Educ. Pract. Vet.*, 15, 742–748.

van Wyk, J.A., Hoste, H., Kaplan, R.M., and Besier, R.B. (2006) Targeted selective treatment for worm management – how do we sell rational programs to farmers? *Vet. Parasitol.*, 139, 336–346.

Werell, E. (2017) Prevalence of *Strongylus vulgaris*. Veterinary thesis, Department of Biomedical Sciences and Veterinary Public Health, SLU, Sweden.

Wildenburg, G., Darge, K., Knab, J., *et al.* (1994) Lymph-nodes of onchocerciasis patients after treatment with ivermectin – reaction of eosinophil granulocytes and their cationic granule proteins. *Trop. Med. Parasitol.*, 45, 87–96.

Wilkes, E.J.A., McConaghy, F.F., Thompson, R.L., *et al.* (2017) Efficacy of a morantel–abamectin combination for the treatment of resistant ascarids in foals. *Aust. Vet. J.*, 95, 85–88.

Xiao, L., Herd, R.P., and Majewski, G.A. (1994) Comparative efficacy of moxidectin and ivermectin against hypobiotic and encysted cyathostomes and other equine parasites. *Vet. Parasitol.*, 53, 83–90.

8

Anthelmintic Resistance

Anthelmintic resistance is defined as "the loss of treatment efficacy of a given anthelmintic formulation that previously exhibited efficacy against the same parasite species and stage, in the same host animal, at the same dosage, and by the same route of administration". This definition spans several important corollaries: (1) if a drug formulation never had efficacy against the parasite and stage in question, then resistance cannot be inferred; (2) whenever anthelmintics are used in an extra-label manner, no conclusions can be drawn regarding resistance because we have no evidence regarding the expected level of efficacy; (3) resistance occurs in some, but not all, specimens of a given parasite species simultaneously present in a treated horse; and (4) expected levels of efficacy differ for parasite species, stages, and anthelmintic formulations. Thus, various efficacy cut-off values (*e.g.*, 90% versus 95%) may be used to designate a population as resistant.

It should come as no surprise whenever biological organisms develop resistance to drugs that are used to combat them. Rather, this is a perfect example of Darwinian survival of the fittest, and there are countless examples of insects, bacteria, and parasites that have become resistant to the available arsenal of therapeutic chemicals. This chapter will describe current findings about anthelmintic resistance in equine helminth parasites, and will also illustrate some of the mechanisms that lead to resistance development in these worms. Table 8.1 presents an overview of resistance reported in major equine parasites.

Benzimidazoles

Cyathostomins were the first equine parasites to demonstrate resistance to a benzimidazole (BZ) drug. Today, BZ-resistant cyathostomins occur world-wide (Peregrine *et al.*, 2014) and BZ resistance appears to be the rule rather than the exception in managed horses. The geographic distribution of reported BZ resistance in strongyles and ascarids is presented in Figures 8.1 and 8.2. Although a five-day regimen of fenbendazole (FBZ) initially achieved satisfactory efficacy against cyathostomin populations with moderate levels of resistance, recent work illustrates that this regimen now has markedly reduced larvicidal effectiveness against populations of highly resistant worms (Reinemeyer, Prado, and Nielsen, 2015; Bellaw *et al.*, 2018). One study confirmed FBZ resistance in a population of horses when strongyle egg counts were not reduced by a single, adulticidal dose of fenbendazole (5 mg/kg). When a five-day regimen (10 mg/kg) of the same anthelmintic was administered to the same horses, some egg count reduction was observed, but efficacies were generally below 50%. In the same study, the larvicidal efficacy of

Handbook of Equine Parasite Control, Second Edition. Martin K. Nielsen and Craig R. Reinemeyer.
© 2018 John Wiley & Sons, Inc. Published 2018 by John Wiley & Sons, Inc.

Table 8.1 Current status of resistance by major nematode parasites to three anthelmintic classes in managed horse herds.

Drug class	Cyathostomins	Large strongyles	*Parascaris* spp.
Benzimidazoles	Widespread	None	Early indications
Pyrimidines	Common	None	Early indications
Macrocyclic lactones	Early indications	None	Widespread

a five-day regimen was 28.6% and 71.2% against EL$_3$s and LL$_3$/L$_4$s, respectively (Reinemeyer, Prado, and Nielsen, 2015). This was well below the historical efficacies of >97% against both larval categories, and thus a clear demonstration of larvicidal resistance. A second study with a different equine population found very similar larvicidal efficacies (Bellaw *et al.*, 2018). These studies confirm the tenet that anthelmintic resistance cannot be overwhelmed by increasing the dosage or the frequency of treatment. Furthermore, they illustrate that while anthelmintic resistance may initially be detected in adult parasites, it will eventually occur in all parasitic stages of the same parasites affected by the given anthelmintic.

Benzimidazole resistance has never been reported in large strongyles and only a few reports suggest resistance in *Parascaris* spp. (Peregrine *et al.*, 2014). Furthermore, BZs appear to be the most appropriate choice for treatment of *Oxyuris equi* infections (Reinemeyer and Nielsen, 2014). Thus, this drug class may still be used with some confidence against non-cyathostomin nematodes. In general, the benzimidazole group can still be viewed as very useful, albeit against a narrower spectrum of parasites than when it was first marketed.

Pyrimidines

While reports of resistance to pyrimidine anthelmintics are not as numerous as for benzimidazoles, pyrantel salt resistance has been widely reported in cyathostomin populations from across the world (Peregrine *et al.*, 2014). Resistance appears to be pronounced in North America (Kaplan *et al.*, 2004; Smith *et al.*, 2015), but also occurs with increasing frequency in Europe (Traversa *et al.*, 2009; Nielsen *et al.*, 2013). Also, morantel tartrate-resistant small strongyles have been reported in Australia (Rolfe, Dawson, and Holm-Martin, 1998).

Recent studies have reported good efficacy of pyrantel salts against *Parascaris* spp. (Veronesi *et al.*, 2009; Lind and Christensson, 2009; Reinemeyer *et al.*, 2010). However, a few reports have documented that some populations of ascarids in the United States and Australia are resistant to pyrantel (Lyons *et al.*, 2008a; Armstrong *et al.*, 2014). The geographic distribution of resistance reports in cyathostomins and ascarids for pyrantel products is presented in Figures 8.1 and 8.2.

Macrocyclic lactones

Although ivermectin has been the most widely used equine anthelmintic in recent decades, no signs of resistance were reported during its first 20 years on the market. That stellar record was interrupted at the beginning of this century, however, by the first reports of avermectin- and milbemycin-resistant *Parascaris* spp. (Boersema, Eysker, and Nas, 2002; Hearn and Peregrine, 2003). Numerous studies have since confirmed the presence of

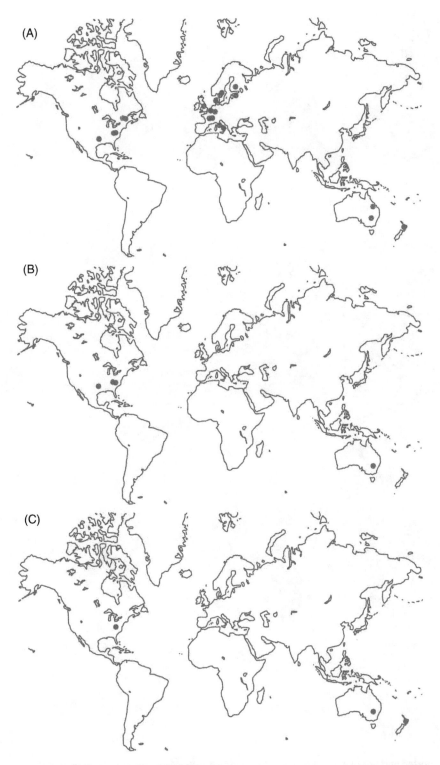

Figure 8.1 Reported findings of anthelmintic resistance in *Parascaris* spp. parasites to (A) macrocyclic lactones, (B) pyrimidines, and (C) benzimidazoles.

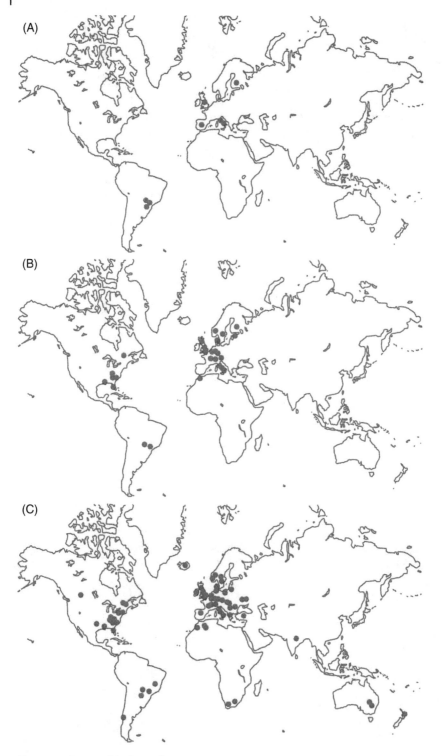

Figure 8.2 Reported findings of anthelmintic resistance in cyathostomin parasites to (A) macrocyclic lactones, (B) pyrimidines, and (C) benzimidazoles.

ivermectin and moxidectin resistance in indigenous populations of *Parascaris* spp. on most continents (Peregrine *et al.*, 2014).

Ivermectin and moxidectin still exhibit good cyathostomin fecal egg count reduction at 14 days post-treatment, and no signs of resistance have been observed among large strongyles. However, several studies have documented that the cyathostomin egg reappearance periods have become shorter after treatment with either compound. Whereas ivermectin and moxidectin historically suppressed egg shedding for 9–13 and 16–22 weeks, respectively, recent studies have reported egg reappearance periods of just four to five weeks for both drugs (Lyons *et al.*, 2008b; 2011; Rossano, Smith, and Lyons, 2010). These observations have been interpreted as early signs of resistance, especially since luminal L_4 stages have been shown to survive treatment at label dosages (Lyons, Tolliver, and Collins, 2009; Lyons *et al.*, 2010; Lyons and Tolliver, 2013; Bellaw *et al.*, 2018).

In recent years, many practitioners have observed evidence of apparent treatment failures of ivermectin against *Oxyuris equi*. These observations were recently confirmed by studies conducted in Germany, France, New Zealand, and the USA (Reinemeyer, 2012; Rock *et al.*, 2013; Wolf, Hermosilla, and Taubert, 2014; Sallé *et al.*, 2016). Thus, ivermectin resistance among *Oxyuris* may be widespread. Similarly, many veterinarians have encountered unprecedented failures of ivermectin to eliminate *Habronema* spp. larval infections in horses with summer sores. The latter observations, however, have not been corroborated in controlled, scientific studies to date.

Other anthelmintics

Apparently, no losses of cestocidal efficacy have been reported for either of the two compounds in common usage, praziquantel or pyrantel pamoate. However, definitive surveys for resistance to cestocides have not been conducted due to a lack of sensitive diagnostic tools. It should be noted that praziquantel resistance has been reported in schistosomes, a parasite group belonging to the flatworm family (Fallon and Doenhoff, 1994). Additionally, an apparent treatment failure of pyrantel pamoate against *Anoplocephala* infection was observed on a farm in Ontario, Canada (Peregrine, Trotz-Williams, and Proudman, 2008). Thus, it should be recognized that cestocidal resistance is at least biologically feasible in equine tapeworms.

Although piperazine is not currently marketed for equine use, it should be mentioned that piperazine resistance has been reported previously in cyathostomins (Drudge *et al.*, 1988).

Mechanisms of anthelmintic resistance

The basic mechanisms behind resistance development deserve some consideration as well. Anthelmintic resistance in helminth parasites differs in a number of ways from antibiotic resistance in bacteria: (1) parasites are eukaryotic and their genes are organized in chromosomes in a manner similar to vertebrates; (2) reproduction is sexual and requires exchange of genetic materials between males and females; (3) generation intervals are comparably much longer, with only one to a few parasite generations per grazing season or calendar year; (4) parasite life cycles involve stages that develop in the environment, where they are minimally exposed to anthelmintics; and (5) similarly, life cycle stages within the host may not be exposed to selection pressures when they occupy sequestered, privileged locations. A pertinent example is found in encysted cyathostomins, which are only exposed to those few drugs with demonstrated larvicidal activity.

The consequence of the last three factors is that only a portion of the parasite population is exposed to an anthelmintic at the time of any treatment. Accordingly, the alleles encoding resistance must accumulate through several successive generations for resistance to achieve clinical significance. Thus, drug resistance develops very slowly in helminths. Apropos to this discussion, ivermectin- and moxidectin-resistant populations of *Parascaris* spp. were not reported until after these products had been used intensively for nearly 20 years (Boersema, Eysker, and Nas, 2002; Hearn and Peregrine, 2003).

An important characteristic of helminth parasites is their incredibly broad genetic diversity. A very wide selection of genes exists within any worm species, and any number of those genes can encode mechanisms that are manifested as anthelmintic resistant. As a fellow parasitologist is fond of saying, "Somewhere in the world, worms exist that are resistant to a class of drugs that has not yet been discovered." In addition to these background genes, recent work with ruminant trichostrongylid parasites has shown that multiple independent mutations occur spontaneously and that a proportion of these mutations confer anthelmintic resistance (Redman *et al.*, 2015). This phenomenon may explain the widespread occurrence of anthelmintic resistance in livestock parasites.

Regardless of origin, the frequency of resistance genes is not likely to increase unless that genetic combination somehow confers an advantage over the rest of the parasite population. Genetic change comes about as a result of factors that are termed selection pressures, and for anthelmintic resistance, the selective advantage is derived from anthelmintic treatment. Whenever a deworming treatment is administered, the ≥99.9% of the population that is susceptible to the drug is removed, and it cannot resume dissemination of its genes until the egg reappearance period expires. Because resistant worms are not killed by the treatment, however, they can continue to reproduce throughout the ERP, in the total absence of their usual competition. In this fashion, the resistant worms are able to contribute more offspring to the population than the average citizen, and the genotypic frequency of resistance factors increases incrementally within the population as a whole.

A number of genes have been identified and associated with anthelmintic resistance to the various drug classes. However, resistance is widely believed to be multigenic, so the few genes identified to date may just be the tip of the iceberg. Hence, anthelmintic resistance is not just a matter of a single point-mutation in the genome, but rather a combination of different genetic determinants. In benzimidazole resistance, for example, specific mutations have been identified in the gene encoding beta-tubulin in cyathostomin parasites (Blackhall, Kuzmina, and von Samson-Himmelstjerna, 2011). The genetic mechanisms are less well understood for other nematocidal drugs. Ivermectin resistance has been associated with changes in genes encoding glutamate-gated chloride channels (GluCl), but this precise mutation does not appear to be very important outside of the laboratory (Beech *et al.*, 2011). Recently, increased expression of P-glycoprotein (Pgp) multidrug transporters has been implicated as having a role in resistance. One isotype of Pgp, Pgp-11, has recently been associated with ivermectin resistance in *Parascaris* spp. (Janssen *et al.*, 2013). Interestingly, this mechanism does not appear to be linked with any particular drug class, so cross-resistance among various drug classes might occur (Beech *et al.*, 2011).

Within a nematode species, the various parasitic life cycle stages often exhibit different susceptibilities to anthelmintics. In general, juvenile and larval stages of strongyles and ascarids are less susceptible than adults, so treatment of a prepatent population may not be as effective as deworming after patency. Pre-adult nematodes are usually the dose-limiting stages for anthelmintic treatment, and resistance is likely to be detected first in juvenile worms. Indeed, the earliest indication of ivermectin and moxidectin resistance in cyathostomins has been the unprecedented survival of fourth stage larvae in the lumen of the gut after treatment (Lyons, Tolliver, and Collins, 2009; Lyons *et al.*, 2010). It does not augur well that luminal L_4 cyathostomins can survive pyrantel treatment, and, indeed, this stage does not appear among the label claims. Lower efficacy against luminal larval stages is suspected for *Parascaris* spp.

It is crucial to recognize that anthelmintic resistance is a permanent, genetic feature of a nematode population. Despite total avoidance of a particular drug class, a parasite population can remain resistant for decades. As a case in point, thiabendazole resistance was induced in a horse band at the University of Kentucky during the 1970s and the affected premises have been occupied by a closed herd for the past 40 years. Yet BZ-resistance was still present at this site after 22 years of rigorous abstention from benzimidazole drugs (Lyons, Tolliver, and Collins, 2007). In another study, benzimidazole-resistant cyathostomins were exposed to bimonthly treatments with pyrantel pamoate for eight years, which resulted in pyrantel resistance, but did not change the underlying benzimidazole resistance status of the worm population (Lyons *et al.*, 2001).

Parasite *refugia*

Parasite *refugia* is a term that refers to any portion of a population that is not exposed to a selection pressure for genetic change. Consequently, a *refugium* func-

tions as a reservoir of susceptible genes. In relation to anthelmintic resistance, parasites in *refugia* are those stages of the life cycle that are not exposed to a drug at the time of deworming. Chapter 3 introduced the term environmental parasite *refugia*, which comprises all nematode stages present on pasture and in fecal piles at any given point in time (*i.e.*, egg, L_1, L_2, L_3). In this section we also consider that proportion of the parasite population that is present in animals that are left untreated, or those parasitic stages that are unaffected by the administered anthelmintic. We sometimes refer to this as animal *refugia*. As one example, encysted cyathostomin larvae are classified as being *in refugia* whenever non-larvicidal anthelmintics are administered.

Refugia have become a central tenet in understanding the development of anthelmintic resistance in parasites (van Wyk, 2001). Because it serves as a reservoir of susceptible genes, maintaining the largest possible *refugia* should minimize selection for anthelmintic resistance. Let us consider this point from another perspective. The only pattern of anthelmintic use that could never result in resistance is complete abstention from deworming. If drugs were never used, then none of the parasite population is exposed, so *refugia* are maximal. Thus, no portion of the population has any selective advantage over another for the opportunity to disseminate their genes.

Whenever a large portion of a worm population is exposed frequently and repeatedly to anthelmintics, the selection pressure for development of resistance is very high. This description fits interval-dosing quite succinctly, especially when larvicidal products are used. If, on the other hand, only 20% of the parasite population is exposed to a drug, the selection for resistant parasites will subsequently be diluted by the 80% *in refugia*. This circumstance reflects what selective treatment approaches are attempting to accomplish. Again, a large *refugium* predicts a slower development of resistance. See Figure 7.1 in the previous chapter for an illustration of this principle.

Now that we understand some basic concepts of parasite *refugia*, we can appreciate another difference between antibiotic resistance in bacteria and anthelmintic resistance in worms. Bacterial populations are rarely *in refugia*, and because they can amplify their numbers within the host, the ratios of animal and environmental *refugia* are reversed from the patterns observed in nematodes.

From Chapter 3, we learned that environmental and climatic factors greatly influence parasite development and transmission, and thus we know that some seasons have larger parasite *refugia* than others (Nielsen *et al.*, 2007). Although L₃s may survive under the snow cover during winter, the relative numbers of larvae ingested during the following spring are much smaller than the numbers ingested during the grazing season. Therefore, treatment when the *refugia* is small (*e.g.*, winter treatments in cold climates) would theoretically increase the selection pressure for anthelmintic resistance. In contrast, cold conditions would likely also prevent parasite transmission due to poor development of free-living stages, so winter treatments may not contribute much to resistance development.

The role of parasite *refugia* in the development of resistance is now a widely accepted concept, but little field evidence has been generated to support it. Field studies with sheep have confirmed its existence (Martin, LeJambre, and Claxton, 1981; Waghorn *et al.*, 2008) and computer models clearly illustrate the importance of unselected populations (Barnes, Dobson, and Barger, 1995). As illustrated in Chapter 7, computer simulations of equine parasites now also further illustrate this principle.

Drug rotation

Rotation among dewormers has long been viewed as a reliable strategy for avoiding anthelmintic resistance. The underlying theory is that parasites resistant to drug "A" will still be susceptible to anthelmintic "B" if it has a different mode of action. Treatment with "B" would remove adults resistant to "A", so the latter would not gain a sustained reproductive advantage. This all sounds very logical, but there is absolutely no evidence to support it. One equine study clearly showed that rotating drugs with each treatment did not appear to slow the development of resistance (Uhlinger and Kristula, 1992). Furthermore, computer modeling with sheep nematodes concluded that rotating drugs does not prevent accumulation of resistant genetic alleles, and therefore does not slow down the development of resistance (Barnes, Dobson, and Barger, 1995). Most recently, similar results have been found for cyathostomin parasites, and one such computer modeling output is presented in Figure 7.2 in the previous chapter. The flaw in the logic is that the resistance alleles are still present in all the environmental stages, so removing adults doesn't eliminate the trait from the population. Further, it appears likely that drug rotation may select for genes such as the P-glycoproteins mentioned earlier in this chapter, which confer resistance across different drug classes.

The resistance problem is further compounded for horses because only three classes of anthelmintics are currently available, and the prevalence of resistance is already high for two of the three. Thus, on many farms, rotation is simply not an option. Many, and perhaps most, horse owners labor under the mistaken notion that the usual complement of anthelmintics is still effective in their herd because they have practiced meticulous rotation in the past. Regardless of the treatment schedule implemented, all anthelmintics employed must be checked routinely to ensure that they still deliver acceptable efficacy. Drug rotation is no substitute for routine testing for anthelmintic resistance on the farm.

References

Armstrong, S.K., Woodgate, R.G., Gough, S., *et al.* (2014) The efficacy of ivermectin, pyrantel and fenbendazole against *Parascaris equorum* infection in foals on farms in Australia. *Vet. Parasitol.*, 205, 575–580.

Barnes, E.H., Dobson, R.J., and Barger, I.A. (1995) Worm control and anthelmintic resistance – adventures with a model. *Parasitol. Today*, 11, 56–63.

Beech, R.N., Skuce, P., Bartley, D.J., *et al.* (2011) Anthelmintic resistance: markers for resistance, or susceptibility? *Parasitology*, 138, 160–174.

Bellaw, J.L., Krebs, K., Reinemeyer, C.R., *et al.* (2018) Anthelmintic therapy of equine cyathostomin nematodes – larvicidal efficacy, egg reappearance period, and drug resistance. *Int. J. Parasitol.*, 48, 97–105.

Blackhall, W.J., Kuzmina, T., and von Samson-Himmelstjerna, G. (2011) Beta-Tubulin genotypes in six species of cyathostomins from anthelmintic-naive Przewalski and benzimidazole-resistant brood horses in Ukraine. *Parasitol. Res.*, 109, 1199–1203.

Boersema, J.H., Eysker, M., and Nas, J.W.M. (2002) Apparent resistance of *Parascaris equorum* to macrocyclic lactones. *Vet. Rec.*, 150, 279–281.

Drudge, J.H., Lyons, E.T., Tolliver, S.C., *et al.* (1988) Piperazine resistance in Population-B equine strongyles – a study of selection in Thoroughbreds in Kentucky from 1966 through 1983. *Am. J. Vet. Res.*, 49, 986–994.

Fallon, P.G. and Doenhoff, M.J. (1994) Drug-resistant schistosomiasis – resistance to praziquantel and oxamniquine induced in *Schistosoma mansoni* in mice is drug-specific. *Am. J. Trop. Med. Hyg.*, 51, 83–88.

Hearn, F.P. and Peregrine, A.S. (2003) Identification of foals infected with *Parascaris equorum* apparently resistant to ivermectin. *J. Am. Vet. Med. Assoc.*, 15, 482–485.

Janssen, I.J.I., Krücken, J., Demeler, J., *et al.* (2013) Genetic variants and increased expression of *Parascaris equorum* P-glycoprotein-11 in populations with decreased ivermectin susceptibility. *PLoS One*, 8, e61635.

Kaplan, R.M., Klei, T.R., Lyons E.T., *et al.* (2004) Prevalence of anthelmintic resistant cyathostomes on horse farms. *J. Am. Vet. Med. Assoc.*, 225, 903–910.

Lind, E.O. and Christensson, D. (2009) Anthelmintic efficacy on *Parascaris equorum* in foals on Swedish studs. *Acta Vet. Scand.*, 51, 45.

Lyons, E.T. and Tolliver, S.C. (2013) Further indication of lowered activity of ivermectin on immature small strongyles in the intestinal lumen of horses on a farm in Central Kentucky. *Parasitol. Res.*, 112, 889–891.

Lyons, E.T., Tolliver, S.C., and Collins, S.S. (2007) Study (1991 to 2001) of drug-resistant Population B small strongyles in critical tests in horses in Kentucky at the termination of a 40-year investigation. *Parasitol. Res.*, 101, 689–701.

Lyons, E.T., Tolliver, S.C., and Collins, S.S. (2009) Probable reason why small strongyle EPG counts are returning "early" after ivermectin treatment of horses on a farm in Central Kentucky. *Parasitol. Res.*, 104, 569–574.

Lyons, E.T., Tolliver, S.C., Drudge, J.H., *et al.* (2001) Continuance of studies on population S benzimidazole-resistant small strongyles in a Shetland pony herd in Kentucky: effect of pyrantel pamoate (1992–1999). *Vet. Parasitol.*, 94, 247–256.

Lyons, E.T., Tolliver, S.C., Ionita, M., and Collins, S.S. (2008a) Evaluation of parasiticidal activity of fenbendazole, ivermectin, oxibendazole, and pyrantel pamoate in horse foals with emphasis on ascarids (*Parascaris equorum*) in field studies on five farms in Central Kentucky in 2007. *Parasitol. Res.*, 103, 287–291.

Lyons, E.T., Tolliver, S.C., Ionita, M., *et al.* (2008b) Field studies indicating reduced activity of ivermectin on small strongyles in horses on a farm in Central Kentucky. *Parasitol. Res.*, 103, 209–215.

Lyons, E.T., Tolliver, S.C., Kuzmina, T.A., and Collins, S.S. (2010) Critical tests evaluating efficacy of moxidectin against small strongyles in horses from a herd for which reduced activity had been found in field tests in Central Kentucky. *Parasitol. Res.*, 107, 1495–1498.

Lyons, E.T., Tolliver, S.C., Collins, S.S., et al. (2011) Field tests demonstrating reduced activity of ivermectin and moxidectin against small strongyles in horses on 14 farms in Central Kentucky in 2007–2009. *Parasitol. Res.*, 108, 355–360.

Martin, P.J., LeJambre, L.F., and Claxton, J.H. (1981) The impact of refugia on the development of thiabendazole resistance in *Haemonchus contortus*. *Int. J. Parasitol.*, 11, 35–41.

Nielsen, M.K., Kaplan, R.M., Thamsborg, S.M., *et al.* (2007) Climatic influences on development and survival of free-living stages of equine strongyles: Implications for worm control strategies and managing anthelmintic resistance. *Vet. J.*, 174, 23–32.

Nielsen, M.K., Vidyashankar, A.N., Hanlon, B.M., *et al.* (2013) Hierarchical model for evaluating pyrantel efficacy against strongyle parasites in horses. *Vet. Parasitol.*, 197, 614–622.

Peregrine, A.P., Trotz-Williams, L., and Proudman, C.J. (2008) Resistance to pyrantel in *Anoplocephala perfoliata* on a Standardbred farm in Canada? *Proceedings, Equine Parasite Drug Resistance Workshop*, Copenhagen, Denmark, July 31–August 1, 2008, pp. 32–33.

Peregrine, A.S., Molento, M.B., Kaplan, R.M., and Nielsen, M.K. (2014) Anthelmintic resistance in important parasites of horses: does it really matter? *Vet. Parasitol.*, 201, 1–8.

Redman, E., Whitelaw, F., Tait, A., *et al.* (2015) The emergence of resistance to the benzimidazole anthelmintics in parasitic nematodes of livestock is characterised by multiple independent hard and soft selective sweeps. *PloS Negl. Trop. Dis.*, 9, e0003494.

Reinemeyer, C.R. (2012) Anthelmintic resistance among non-strongylid parasites of horses. *Vet. Parasitol.*, 185, 9–15.

Reinemeyer, C.R. and Nielsen, M.K. (2014) Review of the biology and control of *Oxyuris equi*. *Equine Vet. Educ.*, 26, 584–591.

Reinemeyer, C.R., Prado, J.C., and Nielsen, M.K. (2015) Comparison of the larvicidal efficacies of moxidectin or a five-day regimen of fenbendazole in horses harbouring cyathostomin populations resistant to the adulticidal dosage of fenbendazole. *Vet. Parasitol.*, 214, 100–107.

Reinemeyer, C.R., Prado, J.C., Nichols, E.C., and Marchiondo, A.A. (2010) Efficacy of pyrantel pamoate against a macrocyclic lactone-resistant isolate of *Parascaris equorum* in horses. *Vet. Parasitol.*, 171, 111–115.

Rock, C., Pomroy, W., Gee, E., and Scott, I. (2013) Macrocyclic lactone resistant *Oxyuris equi* in New Zealand. *Proceedings of 24th International Conference of the WAAVP*, 25–29 August, p. 520.

Rolfe, P.F., Dawson, K.L., and Holm-Martin, M. (1998) Efficacy of moxidectin and other anthelmintics against small strongyles in horses. *Aust. Vet. J.*, 76, 332–334.

Rossano, M.G., Smith, A.R., and Lyons, E.T. (2010) Shortened strongyle-type egg reappearance periods in naturally infected horses treated with moxidectin and failure of a larvicidal dose of fenbendazole to reduce fecal egg counts. *Vet. Parasitol.*, 173, 349–352.

Sallé, G., Cortet, J., Koch, C., *et al.* (2016) Ivermectin failure in the control of *Oxyuris equi* in a herd of ponies in France. *Vet. Parasitol.*, 229, 73–75.

Smith, M.A., Nolan, T.J., Riege, R., *et al.* (2015) Efficacy of major anthelmintics for reduction of fecal shedding of strongyle-type eggs in horses in the Mid-Atlantic region of the United States. *Vet. Parasitol.*, 214, 139–143.

Traversa, D., von Samson-Himmelstjerna, G., Demeler, J., *et al.* (2009) Anthelmintic resistance in cyathostomin populations from horse yards in Italy, United Kingdom and Germany. *Parasite Vector*, 2, S2.

Uhlinger, C.A. and Kristula, M. (1992) Effects of alternation of drug classes on the development of oxibendazole resistance in a herd of horses. *J. Am. Vet. Med. Assoc.*, 201, 51–55.

van Wyk, J.A. (2001) Refugia – overlooked as perhaps the most potent factor concerning the development of anthelmintic resistance. *Onderstepoort J. Vet. Res.*, 68, 55–67.

Veronesi, F., Moretta, I., Moretti, A., *et al.* (2009) Field effectiveness of pyrantel and failure of *Parascaris equorum* egg count reduction following ivermectin treatment in Italian horse farms. *Vet. Parasitol.*, 161, 138–141.

Waghorn, T.S., Leathwick, D.M., Miller, C., and Atkinson, D.S. (2008) Brave or gullible: Testing the concept that leaving susceptible parasites in refugia will slow the development of anthelmintic resistance. *N. Z. Vet. J.*, 56, 185–153.

Wolf, D., Hermosilla, C., and Taubert, A. (2014) *Oxyuris equi*: lack of efficacy in treatment with macrocyclic lactones. *Vet. Parasitol.*, 201, 163–168.

Section III

Diagnosis and Assessment of Parasitologic Information

9

Diagnostic Techniques

Clinical signs of gastrointestinal parasite infection are non-specific and the results of clinical pathology evaluations (*e.g.*, hemogram, serum chemistry) provide only tentative support at best. Parasitic disease is rarely associated with pathognomonic findings, so clinicians are left with pattern recognition. Typical manifestations of parasitism include ill-thrift, a rough haircoat, and pot-bellied appearance. Horses younger than four years of age are more likely to be clinically affected by parasites, and clinical parasitism should always be included among the differential diagnoses for this age group. As described in Chapter 2, gastrointestinal helminthiasis can result in colic and diarrhea, but multiple, alternative differentials for these signs exist as well.

Certain clinical findings lend strong support to a diagnosis of clinical parasitism. Rectal palpation or ultrasound examination of a thickened and dilated cranial mesenteric artery has been used to diagnose *Strongylus vulgaris* infection in small horses (Greatorex, 1977; Wallace *et al.*, 1989).

One of the most useful laboratory parameters is serum protein concentration, which is often reduced in cases of larval cyathostominosis. However, this is not pathognomonic because other gastrointestinal conditions, such as *Lawsonia intracellularis* infection, can cause hypoproteinemia as well. Eosinophilia is classically associated with parasitic migration, but absolute counts are generally inconsistent and difficult to interpret. Therefore, eosinophil counts have no practical diagnostic value.

The majority of currently available tools for the diagnosis of parasitism are based on detection or enumeration of parasite progeny (eggs or larvae) shed in the feces of a horse. Positive findings require the presence of an adult worm population. This methodology has several practical limitations. First, strongylid parasites are most pathogenic during their larval stages, which are sexually immature and not capable of producing eggs. Second, some parasite species, such as the lungworm (*Dictyocaulus arnfieldi*) or liver fluke (*Fasciola hepatica*) may not reach sexual maturity in the horse, and therefore no offspring are produced. Such prepatent or occult parasite infections are very difficult to diagnose. Despite these shortcomings, fecal examination (coprology) remains the cornerstone of equine parasitologic diagnosis.

Identification of parasite reproductive products occurring in equine fecal samples is less complicated than for most domestic animals because the eggs are roughly the same size. As a rule of thumb, most equine parasite eggs approximate the dimensions of a typical strongyle egg (about 50 μm × 100 μm), have a smooth surface, and identifiable contents. Egg-like objects much larger than this, such as mite eggs, are likely artifacts, whereas much smaller

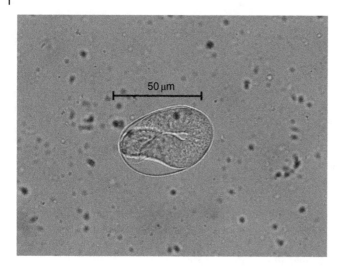

Figure 9.1 Egg of *Strongyloides westeri*.

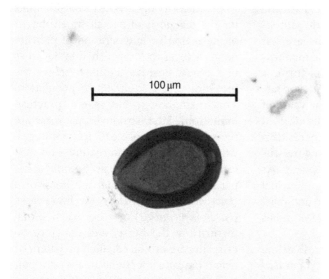

Figure 9.2 Oocyst of *Eimeria leuckarti*.

structures are often pollen grains or other ingested plant material. A few parasites can be identified by the distinct morphology of their eggs. The most unique of these is *Parascaris* spp., which is described further below. Other distinctive parasite eggs include those of *Strongyloides westeri* (Figure 9.1), which are most often identified in foals less than six months of age. Oocysts of the protozoan parasite *Eimeria leuckarti* are unusually large and have a very distinct appearance (Figure 9.2). These are seen almost exclusively in young horses, and even then only infrequently. Occasionally,

eggs of the equine pinworm *Oxyuris equi* may be observed during fecal examination (Figure 9.3), but, as a rule, eggs of this parasite are found around the anus and are not passed in the feces. Eggs of the liver flukes *Fasciola hepatica* or *Dicrocoelium lanceolatum* may be identified rarely. Finally, eggs of Anoplocephalid tapeworms are easily distinguishable when found on fecal examination, but modifications of diagnostic techniques are required to specifically detect tapeworm eggs (see tapeworm diagnostics). We present the main coprologic techniques in this chapter.

Figure 9.3 *Oxyuris equi* egg next to a strongyle egg. Note the operculum at one end (arrow).

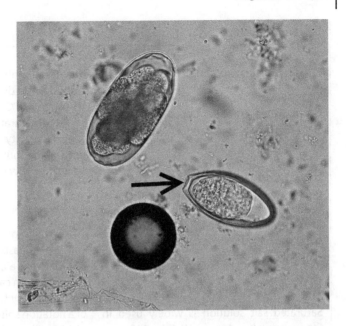

Coprology

Fecal flotation

Although parasite eggs may be present in very large numbers, they nevertheless occupy a relatively small volume of any sample of fecal material. Detection of parasite reproductive products in feces requires physical separation of eggs from the bulk of other organic material present, and subsequent concentration in a relatively small volume for convenient microscopic observation. Helminth eggs have a mass (or specific gravity) that is greater than that of water (s.g. of $H_2O = 1.000$), but lower than most other biological materials present in feces. Equine strongyle eggs typically range from 1.04 to 1.05 in specific gravity while the corresponding values for *A. perfoliata* and *Parascaris* spp. eggs are 1.06–1.07 and 1.08–1.09, respectively (Norris *et al.*, 2017). If feces were mixed with tap water, the eggs would sink along with the majority of the fecal material. If feces were mixed with a dilute solution of some sugar or chemical salt (*e.g.*, sucrose, $NaNO_3$, NaCl, $MgSO_4$, $HgCl_2$) with a specific gravity ≥ 1.18, the helminth eggs would float, but the heavier organic matter would still sink. By transferring such a mixture to a tall cylinder with a relatively small diameter, the floating eggs could be concentrated in a relatively small volume of solution at the very top of the liquid column. This physical isolation of eggs by differences in specific gravity can be expedited by centrifugation. Sidebar 1 contains recipes for two commonly used flotation media.

Fecal flotation is a qualitative technique that can only document the presence or absence of helminth eggs. The lack of standardization of this technique precludes quantitation of egg counts as well as accurate comparisons of egg shedding among horses or in the same horse over time.

Fecal egg counts

Fecal egg counts remain the cornerstone of equine diagnostic parasitology, although recent advances indicate that other methodologies may soon have an important clinical value as well. All egg-counting methods are based on the flotation principle discussed previously. Quantitative techniques differ primarily in that the essential components (feces and flotation solution) are measured carefully, a known representative volume of the mixture is examined,

---

Sidebar 1 Flotation media

Sheather's sugar solution

Sheather's sugar solution is widely used in North American laboratories. Add 454 g (1 lb) of sucrose (table sugar) to 355 ml of very hot water, or stir into steaming water on a hot plate. Stir until dissolved and allow to cool. Sucrose solution will support the growth of mold at room temperature, so keep refrigerated and use quickly or add 6 ml of formaldehyde (37%) for preservation. The specific gravity of Sheather's sugar solution is usually >1.25.

Saturated sugar–salt solution

Saturated salt solution is widely used in European laboratories. Weigh 375 g of glucose monohydrate and 250 g of sodium chloride. Add distilled water q.s. 1 liter total. Warm to 80 °C and stir gently until dissolved. A saturated salt solution will have a specific gravity around 1.18 and can be used alone, but by adding the glucose, a specific gravity of >1.25 can be achieved.

Checking specific gravity

The specific gravity of flotation solutions can be measured with a hydrometer. Alternatively, a carefully measured volume of the solution can be weighed with a sensitive laboratory balance. For example, 10 ml of a flotation solution with a specific gravity of 1.25 will weigh 12.5 grams.

---

and the numbers of parasite reproductive products are counted and recorded. These elements permit calculation of a diagnostic result (fecal egg count) that is expressed in eggs per gram of feces (EPG). Reproductive products of different species of parasites are counted and reported separately.

Numerous fecal egg-counting methods have been described, such as the McMaster (Gordon and Whitlock, 1939), Stoll (Stoll, 1923), and Wisconsin (Cox and Todd, 1962) techniques. Newer methods such as the FECPAK (Presland, Morgan, and Coles, 2005), FLOTAC (Cringoli *et al.*, 2010), and Mini-FLOTAC (Barda *et al.*, 2013) techniques are basically derivations of the McMaster test. The various methods differ primarily in how the quantity of feces is measured and how the eggs are isolated for counting. Some techniques employ passive flotation (Gordon and Whitlock, 1939; Presland, Morgan, and Coles, 2005; Barda *et al.*, 2013) and other methods require the use of a centrifuge (*e.g.*, Cox and Todd, 1962; Roepstorff and Nansen, 1998; Cringoli *et al.*, 2010), and are inherently more time-consuming.

Several parameters are important to consider in assessing the applicability of a given egg-counting technique. These include limit of detection, accuracy, precision, sensitivity, and specificity. Positive and negative predictive values can be useful as well, if they are available. The current section will summarize the interpretation of each of these parameters when assessing a given egg-counting technique.

Limit of detection

The limit of detection is defined as the lowest, positive fecal egg count (FEC) that can be reported by a certain technique. Most quantitative methods are essentially dilution techniques. One counts the number of eggs in a representative sample of feces and mathematically extrapolates the number of eggs counted to a standard reporting unit (usually eggs per gram, EPG). These calculations require that the number of counted eggs be multiplied by a factor that is determined by the amount of feces processed, the volume of fluid in which it is suspended, and the volume of subsample that is subsequently analyzed and counted. This multiplication factor and the limit of detection should be identical, because the lowest positive egg count is 1 EPG. The limit of detection is of importance when analyzing samples containing low numbers of eggs. A common example would be analysis of samples collected after anthelmintic treatment to assess therapeutic efficacy (see Chapter 10). An egg-counting technique with a limit of detection of 25 eggs per gram, for instance, would not give the same numerical results as a method with a sensitivity of 1 egg per gram. As an example, if the "true" egg count for a given sample were 17 eggs per gram, the former technique, with a limit of detection of 25 eggs per gram, could yield a result of "0" EPG. This number should not be interpreted literally that no eggs were present, but rather that the true number was lower than the limit of detection (*i.e.*, <25 EPG). Sidebars 2 and 3 present examples of two egg-counting techniques with different limits of detection.

Sidebar 2 A simple McMaster egg count technique

This is a simple McMaster method for routine application in veterinary practice. This technique does not require centrifugation and has a limit of detection of 25 EPG.

Materials

Disposable cups, wooden tongue depressors, disposable plastic pipettes, laboratory balance (scale) with 0.1 gram accuracy, cheese cloth (17 thread), McMaster counting chamber, flotation solution with a specific gravity in the range of 1.18 to 1.25 (ZnSO$_4$, saturated salt, saturated sugar–salt, or Sheather's sugar), compound microscope.

1) Weigh out 4 g of feces in a small container or paper cup.
2) Add 26 ml of flotation medium (to bring the volume up to 30 ml) to feces. Mix well.
   a) Note: If you do not have a scale, you can add feces to the 26 ml of solution and when the volume reaches 30 ml, you have added 4 g.
3) Strain through one or two layers of cheesecloth, one layered gauze squares, or tea strainer), mix well.
4) Mix the sample well and then immediately withdraw about 1 ml of the suspension with a pipette or syringe and fill the first counting chamber of the McMaster slide.
   a) Repeat the process to fill the second chamber.
   b) Let the slide stand for two to five minutes to allow the eggs to float to top.
   i) If grossly visible air bubbles are present, the chamber should be emptied and refilled.
5) Steps 3 and 4 should be done at the same time without letting the sample sit between steps, since the eggs are in a flotation fluid and will immediately begin to rise to the top of the fluid. You want to be sure to get a representative sample of the mixed solution.
6) Once chambers are filled, step 3 can be started for the next sample.
7) Once filled, the chambers can set for 60 minutes before counting without causing problems if using sodium nitrate. Longer than this and drying/crystal formation can begin. With sodium chloride, crystal formation occurs much more quickly.
8) Count all eggs inside of grid areas (only count the eggs that have more than half of their area inside the outer lines of the grid) at 100× total magnification (10× ocular lens and 10× objective lens). Focus on the top layer, which contains the very small air bubbles (small black circles). Count both chambers.
   a) Count only strongyle eggs. Ascarid, *Strongyloides*, and tapeworm eggs, and *Eimeria* oocysts can also be counted, but should be counted separately from the strongyle eggs.
9) Multiply the number of counted eggs in each category by 25 to achieve the number of eggs per gram (EPG) per egg type.

The limits of detection of the quantitative fecal examination tests listed previously range from one to 100 EPG. An egg count technique with a high limit of detection (*e.g.*, 100 EPG) is not necessarily inferior to one that has a very low limit of detection. Tests with high limits of detection (*i.e.*, ≥25 EPG) are far less labor-intensive and they are just as reliable for identifying high egg shedders in a herd. Differences in precision and sensitivity between methods are merely academic when results engender the same management decision.

Accuracy and precision

As parasite egg counts can be notoriously variable, accuracy and precision are arguably the most important parameters to consider when deciding on a given method. "Accuracy" is defined as the ability of a test to measure as close to the true egg count as possible, whereas "precision" is a measure of repeatability, *i.e.*, how similar repeated counts on the same sample will be to each other. It is important to recognize that accuracy and precision are not synonyms as they actually mean different things. Traditionally, these parameters have not been measured in the world of veterinary parasitology, but they have been adopted in many recent publications.

In general, better precision can be achieved by increasing the volume of fecal material examined microscopically. This attribute has been achieved successfully with the FLOTAC technique, in which the counting chamber accommodates 10 ml. Similarly, the chambers of the Mini-FLOTAC device hold 1 ml, as opposed to 0.3 ml in the classical McMaster chamber, and this greater volume examined achieves substantially higher precision (Noel *et al.*, 2017). Running repeated samples from the same sample is another way to increase the volume examined and improve precision. Exercising strict adherence to the egg-counting protocol, regularly cleaning of microscope lenses and ensuring that personnel are properly trained will all contribute to reduced variability and, hence, improved precision.

Accuracy depends on several factors that represent potential sources of egg loss during processing. One way to optimize accuracy is to ensure thorough homogenization of the fecal suspension prior to subsampling and counting eggs. For example, the Mini-FLOTAC system includes a homogenizer that can effectively suspend the sample and facilitate liberation of eggs for flotation. As a result, the Mini-FLOTAC technique has performed more accurately than the McMaster technique (Noel *et al.*, 2017).

Diagnostic sensitivity and specificity

Sensitivity and specificity are the classic diagnostic parameters used to assess the value and reliability of a diagnostic test, and they remain important for parasite egg counting techniques as well. They are less relevant than accuracy and precision, however, because they only pertain to the qualitative aspects of the given technique, *i.e.*, the ability to correctly identify positive and negative samples. As mentioned above, these aspects are mostly important when analyzing samples with low egg counts. Diagnostic sensitivity could be confused with the limit of detection described above, because the two are clearly related. A lower limit of detection is likely to return more positive samples and thus increase the diagnostic sensitivity. Therefore a good rule of thumb is that techniques with lower limits of detection often offer better diagnostic sensitivity than techniques with higher limits of detection. Newer procedures like the FLOTAC and Mini-FLOTAC both have superior sensitivity compared to the McMaster and Wisconsin techniques (Cringoli *et al.*, 2010; Noel *et al.*, 2017).

Positive and negative predictive values

While not often reported in veterinary medicine, positive and negative predictive values are more relevant to a practice situation than sensitivity and specificity. While sensitivity is the measure of the proportion of true positive samples that give a positive test result with the given technique, the positive predictive value is the proportion of samples with positive test results that accurately represent truly infected horses. The true status of a given sample (*i.e.*, gold standard information) is never available to us in a practice setting, which makes the sensitivity/specificity calculations somewhat backward. The predictive values, on the other hand, are more straightforward as they basically tell us the likelihood of a given test result (positive or negative) being correct.

A fecal egg count performed by someone capable of recognizing a parasite egg generally has a high positive predictive value (Nielsen *et al.*, 2010b), so a positive egg count means infection. However, negative predictive values are usually lower, meaning that horses with negative egg counts can still harbor worms (Nielsen *et al.*, 2010b). A recent study comparing the Mini-FLOTAC and McMaster techniques found both to have positive predictive values above 95%. However, the Mini-FLOTAC had a negative predictive value of 85% compared to 69% for McMaster (Noel *et al.*, 2017). This difference can be ascribed to the lower limit of detection for Mini-FLOTAC compared to McMaster (5 EPG versus 50 EPG), with the result that greater proportions of low egg-count samples are not detected by the McMaster method.

Diagnostic parameters summarized

The take-home message from this discussion is that egg-counting techniques with lower limits of detection usually have superior scores for precision and a negative predictive value. The McMaster technique is widely used in veterinary practice because it is simple and relatively user-friendly, but it has relatively high limits of detection (often 25 EPG or above). This means that the negative predictive value and method precision are both likely to be lower than more refined methods. These differences have relevant implications for interpreting fecal egg count reduction tests (see Chapter 10). However, the McMaster technique remains very useful for identifying high strongyle egg shedders. The Wisconsin technique offers very low limits of detection (down to 1 EPG), which provides a strong negative predictive value, but the quantity of feces examined is usually very small, which compromises the Wisconsin's precision (Sidebar 3). The FLOTAC and Mini-FLOTAC techniques mentioned above offer excellent diagnostic parameters, but have only been used for research purposes thus far and are therefore not yet available to equine practitioners and their clients.

The choice of egg-counting technique in practice should depend on whether the aim is to primarily identify moderate and high strongyle shedders, for which the lower limit of detection is less important, or to conduct a fecal egg-count reduction test, wherein sensitivity, precision, and limit of detection are all very important. Furthermore, practical and pragmatic considerations need to be made as well. Is a functional microscope with clean objectives available and is an adequate centrifuge with a swing bucket rotor at hand? Finally, have the personnel been adequately trained in performing the technique? Table 9.1 summarizes some key parameters to consider when choosing a fecal egg-counting technique.

It is often claimed that egg counts from the same horse can vary significantly during the day and that even more variability can be expected between consecutive days. Although variability can be substantial, these statements are not supported by

Sidebar 3 Modified Wisconsin sugar flotation method

The Modified Wisconsin method is an example of a very sensitive egg counting technique, with a limit of detection of one egg per gram (EPG). As opposed to the McMaster technique, this method requires a centrifuge.

Materials

Disposable cups, pipette or syringe, wooden tongue depressors, laboratory balance with 0.1 gram accuracy, cheese cloth (17 thread), funnel, Sheather's solution, microscope slides, cover slips (18mm×18mm), centrifuge, microscope.

1) Weigh out 1 g of fecal sample in a small beaker (50–100 ml).
2) Add 20 ml of tap water to the fecal material.
3) Stir very well with a spatula and mash the material until it is completely broken apart.
4) Pour the mixture through the funnel with one layer of cheesecloth (or tea strainer) into another beaker (150–250 ml), stirring the material in the funnel while pouring. Press the material remaining in the funnel with the spatula until nearly dry.
5) Add 10 ml of tap water to the beaker and rinse into a mixture the material clinging to the sides and bottom, and then pour this mixture through the material in the funnel, stirring the material in the funnel while pouring. Press the material in the funnel until dry again and then discard.

6) Stir the material in the beaker and immediately pour the contents of the beaker into two 15 ml tubes, being careful to divide it as equally as possible. There should not be any material left in the beaker.
7) Centrifuge the tubes for 5 to 7 minutes at 300 g to pull fecal debris to the bottom of the tube.
8) Pour off the supernatant, leaving the pellet at the bottom of the tubes.
9) Fill the tubes to just over the top with Sheather's solution and place a cover slip on to the meniscus.
10) Centrifuge at 300 g for 10 minutes.
    a) Note that if a swing-bucket rotor is not available then a fixed-angle rotor can be used, but cover slips may fall off. If using a fixed-angle rotor the procedure should be modified as follows: the tube is initially filled only ¾ full with Sheather's solution and then centrifuged. Each tube is transferred to a rack (to position vertically) and filled with Sheather's solution until a positive meniscus forms. Then a coverslip is placed on the tube and the tube is left to sit for 10–15 minutes before removing the coverslip and placing it on a slide for counting.
11) Let sit for about 5 minutes, and then remove the cover slip and place on a slide.
12) Examine the entire cover slip from both tubes and count the number of eggs that you find.
13) The number of eggs counted equals the EPG as the detection limit is 1 EPG.

Table 9.1 Summary of various egg-counting techniques used in horses. These are rated with respect to diagnostic performance as well as practical aspects discussed in Chapter 9.

Technique	Limit of detection*	Precision	Accuracy	Sensitivity	Specificity	Centrifugation	Time consumption
McMaster	25–50	Low	Low	Low	High	No	Low
Wisconsin	1–5	Low	Low	Moderate	High	Yes	High
FLOTAC	1	High	High	High	High	Yes	High
Mini-FLOTAC	5–10	Moderate	High	Moderate	High	No	Moderate

*Limit of detection is expressed in eggs per gram (EPG).

research data. In one study, six horses with different strongyle FECs were sampled at regular, six-hour intervals for five consecutive days. Three subsamples were prepared from each sample and three egg counts were performed from each subsample. This study found no variance among time points during the five days and only 0.09% of the variance was due to daily differences. The overwhelming majority of the variance in this data set was found between subsamples and between repeated counts from the same sample (Carstensen *et al.*, 2013). The take-home message from this study is that the main source of variation between repeated egg counts is due to the distribution of eggs within the fecal sample.

A simple way to improve the diagnostic performance of the McMaster technique is to simply count more chambers or to count the entire chamber instead of just the area under the grid (Lester and Matthews, 2014). This modification increases the volume examined and thus lowers the limit of detection, which again would have a positive impact on negative predictive value and precision. However, this clearly requires more technician time, so one must evaluate whether the added value is justified by the intended purpose of the egg counts in each situation.

In general, fecal egg counts can be used for three purposes: (1) as a diagnostic tool for clinical cases; (2) as a surveillance tool for identifying high egg shedders; and (3) to conduct fecal egg-count reduction testing (FECRT). It is important to recognize that FEC results are not equally useful for these three purposes. The following discussion will address these applications individually.

Clinical diagnostic tool

Overall, the clinical implications of FEC results should be interpreted with great caution, primarily because cyathostomin infections are ubiquitous but generally not very pathogenic. Therefore, the mere presence of strongyle eggs in the feces has little diagnostic value. Second, it should be remembered that prepatent larval phases are generally more pathogenic than adult worms, so a zero egg count does not rule out parasitic disease. Lastly, egg counts have no direct correlation with the size of the worm burden, as demonstrated in one retrospective study (Nielsen *et al.*, 2010b). Furthermore, as mentioned previously, FECs generally have a low negative predictive value (NPV), so an FEC result of zero does not guarantee the absence of mature worm populations.

In summary, FECs have no value as a clinical diagnostic tool, and treatments should be based on the clinical presentation, history, and diagnostic findings other than the FEC.

FEC as a surveillance tool

When FECs are used as a means of strongyle surveillance, the main purpose is not to detect adult worms in the horse or to estimate their numbers, but rather to characterize the level of environmental contamination originating from that animal. This parameter has been termed the Strongyle Contaminative Potential (SCP).

Several studies have shown that adult horses tend to maintain roughly similar levels of egg output over time (Nielsen, Haaning, and Olsen, 2006; Becher *et al.*, 2010). This phenomenon appears to be particularly pronounced in horses with a low SCP, *i.e.*, those that consistently shed relatively few eggs. Horses with 0 or very low egg counts often maintain this level of egg shedding throughout their adult lives, even in the absence of anthelmintic treatment. Low shedders comprise 40–60% of most adult horse populations. A smaller proportion (perhaps 20–30%) of adult horses in a herd shed moderate numbers of eggs, as depicted in Figure 9.4. A minor portion of the herd (10 to 30%) can be classified as high shedders, and they are responsible for more environmental

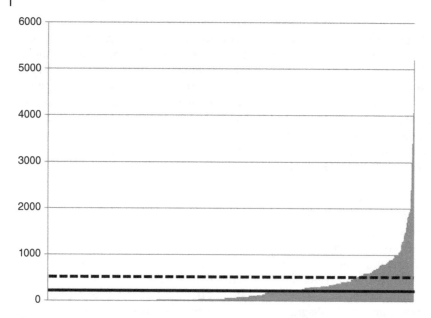

Figure 9.4 Typical distribution of strongyle egg counts in horses. Data from 1566 adult horses on 64 different premises in Denmark. Approximately 60% of horses were shedding <200 EPG (bold horizontal line), but these only contributed 11% of the total numbers of eggs produced. Another 24% of horses were shedding between 200 and 500 EPG (between dashed and bold lines), corresponding to ~25% of the eggs passed. The remainder of horses (only ~15%) had egg counts >500 EPG, but they contributed 64% of the total eggs shed.

contamination with worm eggs than the other two categories combined. In fact, it has been estimated that 80% of all the strongyle eggs passed by a herd originate from only 10 to 20% of herd members (Kaplan and Nielsen, 2010; Relf *et al.*, 2013; Lester *et al.*, 2013).

The consistency of the magnitude of egg shedding is illustrated with farm records in Table 9.2. In this data set, 424 horses were sampled in the spring and fall of three consecutive years. Horses received anthelmintic treatments only when their FEC was 200 EPG or above. The table clearly illustrates the strong tendency of egg counts from horses with low SCP to remain low over time. This phenomenon provides the basis for selective therapy regimens in which horses with the lowest levels of egg shedding are left untreated. It is important to emphasize that this approach can only be applied to adult

Table 9.2 Consistency of fecal egg count levels in individual horses over time. In this study, 424 horses were analyzed twice yearly, in spring and autumn, for three consecutive years. Horses received anthelmintic treatment if their egg counts were 200 EPG or higher. The table predicts the outcome of a subsequent fecal egg count, when the results of two previous sampling occasions were known.

Result of two previous egg counts	Result of third egg count	Probability (%)
0, 0	0	82
0, 0	<200	91
<200, <200	<200	84
≥200, ≥200	≥200	59

Source: Reprinted from Veterinary Parasitology, 135, Nielsen, M.K., Haaning, N., and Olsen, S.N., Strongyle egg shedding consistency in horses on farms using selective therapy in Denmark, pp. 333–335, Copyright (2006), with permission from Elsevier.

horses. The principle of selective therapy is described further in Chapter 7.

As mentioned in previous sections, egg counts have considerable variability, and one should not expect identical results for repeated egg counts, even if using multiple samples from the same fecal ball. As a rule of thumb, the variability of any given egg count is ~50% (Uhlinger, 1993). In other words, an FEC result of 1000 EPG represents a potential range of 500–1500 EPG. Thus, a quantitative result for a horse with a "true" moderate egg count might occasionally fall into the low range and that animal would remain untreated if the decision were based on a single egg count. However, from a herd perspective, the overall reduction of egg output would not be affected significantly if a few horses with marginal egg counts were misclassified as low or moderate shedders. If more precise results are warranted, however, egg counts from the same sample can be repeated and a mean value calculated. Alternately, a technique with greater precision could be chosen for determining egg counts.

Routine laboratory screening can be applied to classify horses as low, moderate, or high strongyle egg shedders. Low shedders generally have egg counts below the predetermined cut-off value for treatment (usually in the 100–500 EPG range) and high shedders typically exhibit more than 500–1000 EPG. Restricting treatment to horses with higher egg counts effectively provides overall reduction of egg shedding by the herd, and simultaneously diminishes the selection pressure for anthelmintic resistance (see Chapter 7 for a discussion of selective therapy).

Early studies in Great Britain demonstrated that strongyle egg shedding also exhibits seasonal variations (Poynter, 1954; Duncan, 1974). In a northern temperate climate, egg counts were markedly lower during winter, even in the absence of anthelmintic treatment. Over the spring months, a gradual increase was observed

from late winter to early summer. This pattern (termed "spring rise") is another example of how parasites spend their resources wisely. Because environmental conditions are unfavorable for egg hatching and larval development during winter, it is not a biologically efficient strategy to pass high numbers of eggs in those months. It is possible that a similar pattern can be observed during summer months in warmer climates. Altogether, this suggests that parasite transmission is synchronized with the grazing season and that parasite monitoring and therapeutic interventions should be applied concurrently. A frequent misinterpretation of this recommendation is that egg counts are less reliable during winter months. Although egg counts may be lower, it does not make them less reliable because this is an accurate reflection of seasonal patterns. We have no evidence to suggest that any of the diagnostic parameters discussed earlier in this chapter are affected by seasonality.

For reliable results, fecal samples should be collected and stored appropriately to reduce variability. Fecal samples should be collected when fresh, if possible. However, studies have shown that samples collected from the stall floor are reliable for the first 12 hours after defecation in both relatively cool (12–17°C) and warm (25–29°C) conditions, when egg counts were performed immediately after collection without further storage (Nielsen *et al.*, 2010a). Airtight storage appears to be critical because egg hatching is an aerobic process, and the minimal availability of oxygen in an airtight container will help to preserve the eggs for flotation. Samples kept in airtight plastic bags at room temperature were reliable for the first 24 hours, but counts declined significantly thereafter. Refrigeration plus airtight storage will maintain reliable samples for at least five days, and perhaps considerably longer (Nielsen *et al.*, 2010a). Freezing fecal samples reduced egg counts by 20 to

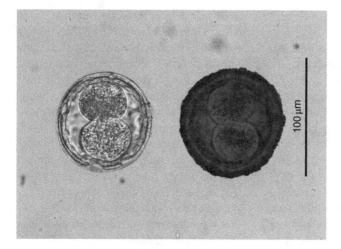

Figure 9.5 Two eggs of *Parascaris* spp. The lighter egg on the left has shed its proteinaceous capsule, a common finding, which is observed in about 10% of eggs encountered in fecal samples.

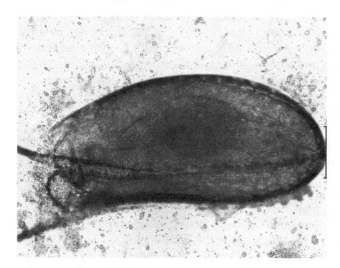

Figure 9.6 Ciliate cysts occur normally in equine fecal samples and are often similar in size to strongyle eggs but have an irregular outline (sizebar = 20 μm).

30% during the initial 24 hours, but no further egg loss was observed after an additional four days. Egg counts quickly declined during storage at 38 °C (100 °F) (Nielsen *et al.*, 2010a).

Interpretation of FECs for foals and weanlings is a complicated proposition because they can harbor *Parascaris* spp. as well as strongyles. A quantitative or qualitative examination technique will yield this information, as both types of eggs are very easy to identify (Figure 9.5). Given findings of anthelmintic resistance in both strongyles and ascarids (see Chapter 8), the choice of anthelmintic may depend on whether strongyle or ascarid eggs are more dominant.

Artifacts in fecal samples can sometimes be misidentified by technical personnel who are unfamiliar with equine samples. Pollen grains, mite eggs, and various naturally occurring ciliate protozoa are occasionally mistaken for parasitic progeny (Figure 9.6).

Detecting anthelmintic resistance

Using fecal egg counts to detect anthelmintic resistance is addressed in Chapter 10 (see Fecal Egg Count Reduction Testing).

Fecal egg-count summary

Fecal egg counts are poor clinical diagnostic tools. They reflect only the presence of adult parasite populations, but not pathogenic larval stages. A negative predictive value is modest, implying a risk of false-negative results. Above 500 EPG, the absolute magnitude of an egg count is not correlated to the size of the adult strongyle worm burden. Despite these limitations, routine FECs are recommended on every horse farm for two purposes: evaluation of anthelmintic efficacy and identification of low, moderate, and high egg shedders for a tailored control strategy.

It is recommended that laboratories performing fecal egg counts routinely validate their techniques against findings by established laboratories.

Baermann technique

The Baermann technique is used to recover live parasite larvae from a fecal sample. Typically, the fecal sample is placed in lukewarm tap water for 24 hours. In an aqueous medium, larvae will swim out of the feces and into the water. Because many larvae tend to be positively geotropic (*i.e.*, swim towards gravity), they congregate in the bottom of a container, wherefrom they can be collected and examined. The use of cylindrical or funnel-shaped flasks concentrates geotropic larvae in a minimal volume of sediment. The Baermann technique has three potential applications in equine parasitology:

1) Detection of *Dictyocaulus arnfieldi* (lungworm) first stage (L_1) larvae. However, as described in Chapter 1, lungworms are primarily found in donkeys and rarely reach sexual maturity in horses. Therefore, a Baermann procedure is not very useful for horses, but can be applied to donkeys.

2) Recovery of cyathostomin larvae that recently emerged from the mucosal membranes of horses with suspected larval cyathostominosis (Olsen *et al.*, 2003). This technique is applicable only to very fresh post-mortem specimens and requires some training to distinguish between the L_4/L_5 larvae emerging from cysts and L_1 or L_2 larvae that hatched during sedimentation at room temperature (see Figure 9.7). This method has not yet been thoroughly validated, but in one author's experience (MKN) false negatives can occur in cases of larval cyathostominosis.

3) Harvest of third stage larvae after coproculture. See below.

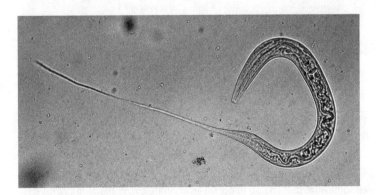

Figure 9.7 Second stage strongyle larva (L_2) harvested from a Baermann apparatus. Note the characteristic whiplash tail.

Larval cultures

Strongyle eggs are very similar in morphology and generally cannot be identified to the genus or species level. Although subtle differences have been reported among first (L_1) and second (L_2) stage larvae (Ogbourne, 1971), diagnoses are never based on examination of these stages. Third stage larvae (L_3), however, have more distinct morphologic characteristics that allow several strongyle species or genera to be identified (Russell, 1948; Bevilaqua, Rodrigues, and Concordet, 1993). Culturing of feces (coproculture) and subsequent identification of L_3s have practical applications both in research and in practice.

All coproculture techniques essentially incubate feces aerobically near room temperature for periods of up to two weeks. Feces can be mixed with an inert material like vermiculite, sphagnum moss, or granular charcoal to delay evaporation and to facilitate oxygenation, but the consistency of equine feces makes it an excellent culture medium even without additives. During the culture period, samples should be monitored daily for desiccation and supplemental water added if needed. Exposure to direct sunlight should be avoided.

Larvae that hatch from eggs in this medium and develop to the L_3 stage are harvested by the Baermann technique. All strongylid larval stages (L_1, L_2, L_3) exhibit a characteristic whiplash tail (Figures 9.7, 9.8, 9.9, and 9.10), but only the L_3s have a double-layered cuticle (larval sheath) and distinct intestinal cells (Figures 9.8, 9.9, and 9.10). *Strongylus vulgaris* larvae are the most readily distinguishable because they possess a high number (28–32) of distinct intestinal cells (Figure 9.8) and are often 50–100% larger than larvae of other

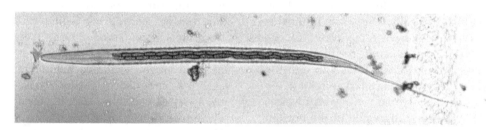

Figure 9.8 Third stage larva (L_3) of *Strongylus vulgaris*. The larva can be identified to species level based on the presence of 28–32 distinct intestinal cells. (*Source*: Photograph courtesy of Jennifer L. Bellaw).

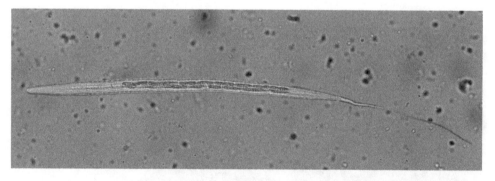

Figure 9.9 The intestinal cells in third stage (L_3) larvae of *Strongylus edentatus* are slender, elongated, and ill-defined, which makes it somewhat challenging to obtain an accurate count. *Triodontophorus* spp. larvae also have 18–20 intestinal cells, but they are well defined and more rectangular. (*Source*: Photograph courtesy of Jennifer L. Bellaw).

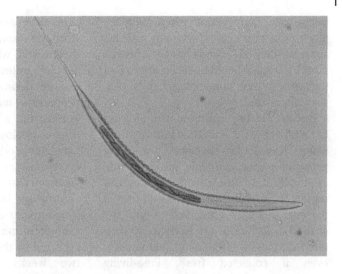

Figure 9.10 Third stage cyathostomin larva (L₃). Note the eight intestinal cells arranged in one row and the double-layered cuticle characteristic of this stage. (*Source*: Photograph courtesy of Jennifer L. Bellaw).

species. No other strongyle larvae exhibit more than 20 cells, but several have 16 to 20 intestinal cells. Consequently, *S. edentatus* (Figure 9.9) must be distinguished from *Triodontophorus* spp. (Strongylinae), *S. equinus* from *Poteriostomum* spp. (Cyathostominae), and *Oesophagodontus robustus* (Strongylinae) from *Trichostrongylus axei* (Trichostrongylidae) by means of intestinal cell shape and other morphologic characteristics (Russell, 1948; Bevilaqua, Rodrigues, and Concordet, 1993). With the exceptions of *Poteriostomum* spp. (16 cells) and *Gyalocephalus capitatus* (12 cells), cyathostomin species all have eight intestinal cells and are easily distinguished from *Strongylus* species, but not from each other. Although some investigators have been able to subdivide eight-cell cyathostomin larvae into subgroups based on morphometric characteristics (Kornas *et al.*, 2009; Bevilaqua, Rodrigues, and Concordet, 1993), the most important practical reason for performing larval cultures is to detect the presence of *S. vulgaris*.

To screen routinely for *S. vulgaris*, practitioners might consider pooling samples from several horses into one culture. However, *S. vulgaris* contributes a very small percentage of the strongyle eggs shed on most farms, and infections can easily be overlooked when samples are pooled (Bracken *et al.*, 2012). Any larval culture will be dominated by cyathostomin larvae, which are easily recognized (Figure 9.10), and large strongyle species often comprise ≤1% of larvae recovered (Bellaw and Nielsen, 2015).

A recent study used historical data to validate larval culturing for diagnosis of infection with two species of large strongyles (Nielsen *et al.*, 2010b). Coproculture foretold the presence of *S. vulgaris* and *S. edentatus* adults at necropsy with a high, positive predictive value. Larval culture yielded occasional false-negative results for both species, however, and had moderate negative predictive values. No linear correlation was observed between counts of larvae per gram of feces (LPG) and adult worm burdens.

Lugol's iodine solution is routinely used to kill larvae and to improve the visibility of intestinal cells before examining the sample microscopically. Lugol's halts the motility of larvae, but will make intestinal cells indistinguishable after about five minutes, thus making identification to species or genus impossible. Chilling larvae by holding microscope slides on a cold thermal block also diminishes motility, but larvae are quickly reactivated by heat from the microscope lamp. Heat inactivation by placing slides on a ~50 °C warming plate for approximately 30 seconds has been proven useful, but care should be taken not to boil the larvae as their morphology can be substantially altered.

Perhaps the most common complication of larval culture is contamination by free-living nematodes. Because free-living nematodes may complete an entire life cycle within a culture medium, they can rapidly overwhelm the parasitic larvae present. Samples collected from the ground or stall floor are likely to be contaminated with free-living nematodes, even if collected fresh. Free-living nematodes are easy to distinguish from strongyle larvae; they lack the typical sheath and whiplash tail, and have no distinct intestinal cells. Many sizes and developmental stages of free-living nematodes may be present, including egg-bearing adults (Figure 9.11). Finally, the morphology of the esophagus of free-living nematodes and L_1 and L_2 strongylids is very characteristic (Figure 9.12), and differs from that of L_3 strongyles.

Although larval culture is technically simple to perform, it requires vigilance, is time-consuming, and results cannot be reported to the owner for approximately two weeks after sample collection.

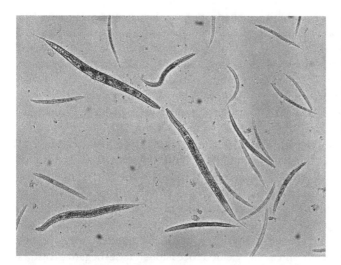

Figure 9.11 Contamination of a larval culture with free-living nematodes. Note the presence of different developmental stages and sizes, as well as the absence of characteristic, long, strongyle tails. (*Source*: Photograph courtesy of Jennifer L. Bellaw).

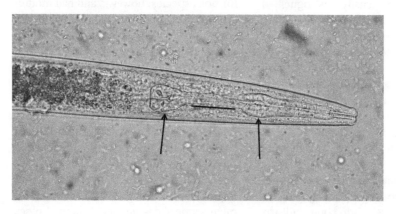

Figure 9.12 Free-living nematodes can be recognized by the shape of the esophagus, which features two bulbs (arrows) separated by a narrow isthmus (straight line). (*Source*: Photograph courtesy of Tina Roust and Maria Rhod).

Because of these practical limitations, molecular diagnostic tools have been investigated to provide more immediate results.

Tapeworm diagnostics

Diagnosing anoplocephalid tapeworm infections remains a challenge despite the utility of several techniques. Fortunately, tapeworm diagnostic methods have been well-validated, so their weaknesses and strengths can be evaluated precisely.

Fecal examination for tapeworm eggs

It is a common misconception that tapeworm proglottids can be readily observed in equine fecal samples. Proglottids of *A. perfoliata* usually disintegrate well before defecation, but should a few remain intact, they would be very hard to see with the naked eye. They measure just a few mm in thickness, and are grayish or brownish in appearance. They do not resemble the off white, rice grain- or cucumber seed-appearance of the proglottids of canine and feline tapeworms. In contrast, proglottids of *A. magna* are much larger (about 0.5 cm × 2 cm), occasionally appear in the feces, and are sometimes observed to be motile.

Similarly, the much smaller proglottids of *Anoplocephaloides mamillana* (about 2 mm × 5 mm) can sometimes be observed intact and motile in the feces.

All diagnostic procedures that rely on detection of tapeworm eggs in feces are compromised by one common factor. Cestodes don't expel eggs at a constant rate, unlike nematode parasites (in fact, tapeworms are hermaphroditic, so there is no division of labor by gender). Rather, tapeworms shed entire body segments, or proglottids, which essentially are bags of eggs. Although proglottids usually disintegrate within the host, the release of eggs from episodic, concentrated sources results in a very uneven distribution of eggs in the feces.

Any qualitative or quantitative fecal examination technique is capable of detecting tapeworm eggs (Figure 9.13), but the sensitivity of most techniques is too low to make a reliable diagnosis. As an example, the diagnostic sensitivity of the simple McMaster technique has been found to be less than 10% for tapeworms (Nielsen, 2016). Thus, if eggs are found, they should be regarded as the tip of the iceberg, and many more could be recovered with a more sensitive and accurate technique.

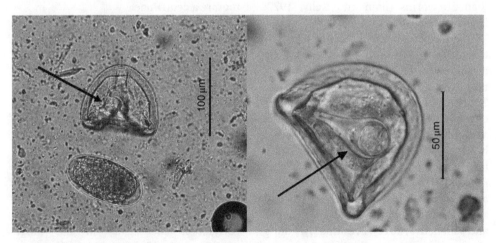

Figure 9.13 Eggs of *Anoplocephala perfoliata*. Eggs often appear D-shaped and contain a distinct onchosphere (pyriform body, arrows). A strongyle egg is included for size comparison on the left panel.

One basic modification employed for detecting tapeworms is to increase the amount of feces examined. Whereas a routine McMaster procedure typically uses 4g of feces, examining 30–40g of feces has been shown to improve the diagnostic sensitivity for tapeworms to about 60% (Nielsen, 2016). Furthermore, the more sensitive tapeworm methods use enhanced flotation with the Stoll or Wisconsin principle, using 10 or 15 ml centrifuge tubes topped with glass cover slips. This accommodation requires a centrifuge with a swing-bucket rotor to prevent cover slips from being dislodged. An example of an egg-counting technique modified for tapeworm detection is presented in Sidebar 4 (Proudman and Edwards, 1992). However, a sensitivity around 60% means there is still a 40% chance of a false-negative result, which should be kept in mind when interpreting these diagnostic results. These likelihoods were based on detection of cestode burdens comprising only a single worm. If the threshold were adjusted to detect 20 or more tapeworms, the sensitivity increases to 90% (Kjær *et al.*, 2007; Proudman and Edwards, 1992). The choice of 20 tapeworms as a cut-off level is supported by the fact that no mucosal pathology is observed with tapeworm burdens of fewer than 20 worms (Bain and Kelly, 1977; Pearson *et al.*, 1993).

One study reported that using concentrated sucrose (s.g. 1.26) as a flotation medium yielded better results than saturated salt or zinc sulfate (Rehbein *et al.*, 2011) and it is likely that similar differences exist between other flotation media as well. Some studies have reported that higher *Anoplocephala* egg counts and a higher percentage of positive samples resulted if fecal samples were collected and examined 24 hours after cestocidal treatment (Sanada *et al.*, 2009; Elsener and Villeneuve, 2011). Presumably, killing the tapeworms resulted in the disintegration of more proglottids within the host gut and thus the release of more eggs into the feces.

It was observed in a Polish study that the proportion of mature *A. perfoliata* tapeworms was highest during the first quarter of the year and that this was statistically associated with higher tapeworm egg counts as well as higher diagnostic sensitivities of a modified fecal egg-counting technique (Tomczuk *et al.*, 2015). These data suggest that the optimal time for tapeworm egg detection would be during winter and early spring in a temperate climate, such as Poland.

A recent study suggested that morphometric measures can be applied to differentiate eggs of *A. perfoliata* and *A. magna*. By measuring the diameter of the oncosphere (see Figure 9.13), it was determined that all *A. perfoliata* eggs examined had oncospheres measuring >15 μm, whereas 97% of *A. magna* eggs were below this threshold (Bohorquez *et al.*, 2014). Such differentiation could have clinical implications because *A. magna* has not been associated with clinical disease.

In summary, the modified egg-count method has proven useful for diagnosing moderate and large tapeworm burdens, while the smaller worm burdens may go undetected. The method is relatively easy to perform in most laboratories, but does require a centrifuge.

Tapeworm serum ELISA

An enzyme-linked immunosorbent assay (ELISA) method is currently available for detection of serum antibodies against 12/13 kDa excretory/secretory (ES) antigens of *Anoplocephala perfoliata*. Diagnostic sensitivity was reportedly in the 68–78% range, whereas specificity levels ranged from 71 to 95% in published studies (Nielsen, 2016). In addition, significant correlations between ELISA results and worm counts have been reported, with correlation coefficients in the range of 0.54–0.63 (Nielsen, 2016). However, interpretation of the results is not as

Sidebar 4 Modified egg counting method for detecting tapeworm eggs

This method is a modification of the Wisconsin technique, because it utilizes centrifugation-enhanced flotation. The key difference is the use of a larger fecal sample to increase the sensitivity of the method. Non-tapeworm parasite eggs will be encountered as well.

Materials

Disposable cups, tap water, wooden tongue depressor, cheesecloth (17 thread), disposable pipettes, 15 ml test tubes, flotation fluid with a specific gravity in the range of 1.18 to 1.25 (such as $ZnSO_4$, saturated salt, $MgSO_4$, saturated sugar–salt, or Sheather's sugar), laboratory balance with 0.1 gram accuracy, microscope slides, cover slips (18 mm × 18 mm).

1) Weigh 30 g of feces in a cup.
2) Add 60 ml of tapwater. Suspend the feces with the tongue depressor and rest for 30 minutes.
3) Stir the suspension and pour through one layer of cheese cloth into another cup. Squeeze the cloth with the spatula to express all liquid into the cup.
4) Pour the fluid into four 15 ml test tubes.
5) Centrifuge for ten minutes at 1000 g.
6) Pour off the supernatant and preserve the pellet. Vortex the pellet (or stir with a wooden applicator stick) to resuspend it in the remaining fluid.
7) Add flotation solution to about 3–5 mm below the rim of the tubes; stir well with a wooden applicator stick.
8) Centrifuge tubes for 5 minutes at 210 g.
9) Transfer tubes to a rack to orient vertically.
10) Gently add flotation solution to the tubes to create a slight meniscus.
11) Place a cover slip on top of each tube and leave for five minutes.
12) One can also fill the entire tube with flotation solution and centrifuge with the cover slips sitting on top of the tubes. However, this requires a centrifuge with a swing-bucket rotor to prevent loss of cover slips during centrifugation.
13) Lift the cover slips off the tubes and place them on one or more microscope slides labeled with the respective horse's ID.
14) Count all tapeworm eggs under the coverslip using the 4× or 10× objective.
15) The total number of tapeworm eggs counted in the four tubes is most often reported without applying a multiplication factor.

straightforward as one might assume. A Danish abattoir study evaluating this assay found higher background levels of antibodies in *A. perfoliata* negative horses, which resulted in a high proportion of false positive results (Kjær *et al.*, 2007). Another study evaluated antibody levels following tapeworm treatment (Abbott *et al.*, 2008) and found that horses remained antibody-positive for up to five months post-treatment. In addition, recent data from horses co-infected with *A. perfoliata* and *A. magna* suggest a lack of species-specificity of the serum antibody ELISA (Bohorquez, Meana, and Luzon, 2012).

These shortcomings are typical for ELISAs and do not indicate any particular issues with these tests. They just indicate that antibody titers reflect exposure rather than contemporaneous infection. The serum ELISA remains a very useful test for investigating historical *Anoplocephala* exposure in a herd, but a positive result for an individual animal may not be a reliable indicator of current infection.

Tapeworm saliva ELISA

Most recently, an ELISA has been developed and validated for detecting antibodies to *A. perfoliata* in saliva samples.

This assay is commercially available in Europe and has a reported sensitivity and specificity of 83% and 85%, respectively (Lightbody, Davis, and Austin, 2016). Preliminary data suggest that the half-life of the measured antibodies is less than for the IgG(T) antibodies measured with the serum ELISA discussed previously. This means that a diagnostic result would convert to negative more rapidly after cestocidal treatment with the saliva test than with a serum ELISA, if the horse does not become re-infected. This assay has the advantage of cost savings over the serum ELISA because horse owners can collect the samples without having to involve a veterinarian. However, given that it measures anticestode antibodies, it still primarily reflects recent exposure rather than actual infection, in a fashion similar to the serum ELISA.

Diagnosis of *Oxyuris equi*

As mentioned in previous chapters, eggs of *Oxyuris equi* are usually not found in the feces due to the egg-laying behavior of the female worms. Irregular patches of eggs, ranging in color from light yellow to pale green and even orange, can be observed in the perianal area. A sample of this material usually contains numerous eggs, but pinworm eggs are often present on infected horses even if no visible deposit is evident.

Two methods are commonly employed to harvest eggs for microscopic examination. In the so-called "Scotch Tape Technique", a piece of clear cellophane tape is applied (sticky side down) to the perianal area and then transferred to a labeled microscope slide. Theoretically, perianal detritus, including *Oxyuris* eggs if present, will adhere to the tape and be captured for inspection. Alternatively, a wooden tongue depressor can be coated lightly with lubricant and then used to firmly scrape the skin surrounding the anus. Material collected will adhere to the lubricant and can be transferred to a microscope slide and distributed for visualization. *Oxyuris* eggs might be present in very low numbers, so detection with either technique may require careful microscopic examination. Given the sequestered anatomic location of oviposition and unlikelihood of environmental contamination, either of these tests should have a very good positive predictive value.

Demonstration of microfilariae

Demonstration of the microfilarial stages of the genera *Onchocerca* and *Parafilaria* is not commonly attempted. However, ante-mortem diagnosis can be accomplished by biopsying a skin sample from an affected area, mincing it into very small pieces, and incubating the sections in tepid saline. Microfilariae can be observed microscopically, swimming within the liquid medium (Klei *et al.*, 1984).

Immunodiagnostics

Although many attempts have been made over the past 20 to 30 years to develop immunodiagnostic assays for the diagnosis of equine helminth infections, very few have been successfully validated. One example is the tapeworm ELISA, mentioned previously, but assays targeting nematode parasites have been less successful.

Elevations of α- and β-globulin fractions and concurrent hypoalbuminemia were observed frequently in mixed strongyle infections (Schultze, Bergfeld, and Wall, 1983; Bailey *et al.*, 1984). However, most protein measurements were found to be non-specific and subject to high degrees of variation, with no pathognomonic pattern for strongyle infection (Bailey *et al.*, 1984; Abbott, Mellor, and Love, 2007). To date, no protein-based diagnostic assay has found application for equine parasite detection in veterinary practice.

A major component of the increased globulin fraction in equine strongyle infections is attributed to antibodies of the IgG(T) subgroup, which have been associated with *Strongylus vulgaris* infection (Patton *et al.*, 1978; Kent, 1987). This finding led to the development of a commercial assay named Aglutinade® Strongyle Test (Virbac), a latex agglutination kit measuring the level of IgG(T) in horse serum (Kent and Blackmore, 1985). Although an association with strongyle infection was observed, other causes of IgG(T) elevation could not be ruled out because specificity of the antibodies was not evaluated. Thus, this assay was found to be of limited value (Klei, 1986) and is no longer marketed. Subsequent attempts were made to develop specific serological assays for IgG(T) antibodies specific against *S. vulgaris*. Despite substantial efforts, cross-reactivity with other nematode species constituted a major obstacle to practical application (Klei *et al.*, 1983; Weiland *et al.*, 1991).

More recently, a serum ELISA was successfully developed and validated for detecting migrating larvae of *S. vulgaris* (Andersen *et al.*, 2013). This assay measures IgG(T) antibodies to a specific protein, rSvSXP, which is produced by migrating larvae. It has been found to perform with a sensitivity and specificity of 73% and 81%, respectively, and a significant, positive correlation was observed to the number of *S. vulgaris* larvae recovered from the mesenteric arteries. Furthermore, the assay appeared to be unaffected by concurrent infection with other parasites, such as cyathostomins and *Parascaris* spp. (Andersen *et al.*, 2013). Recent work with this assay has illustrated that infected animals seroconvert about 60–90 days post-infection and that horses can remain ELISA-positive for up to 5 months following effective anthelmintic treatment (Nielsen *et al.*, 2014; 2015). Thus, this assay should be interpreted in a fashion similar to other antibody ELISAs; a

positive test result may not reflect actual infection, but rather exposure to the parasite within the past five months. This assay is not currently available in veterinary practice.

Fasciola hepatica ELISA

A serum ELISA was developed recently for detecting antibodies to the liver fluke, *Fasciola hepatica*, in horses (Nelis *et al.*, 2009). A positive correlation was shown between ELISA results and elevations of gamma glutamyl transferase (GGT), an enzyme that is regarded as a reliable indicator of bile duct pathology. Unpublished observations by one of the authors (MKN), however, did not find a similar association between GGT elevations and antibody titers using this assay. Further validation will be required before a useful test can be marketed to veterinary practitioners in *Fasciola*-endemic areas.

A recent study assessed the suitability of a commercial copro-antigen ELISA for diagnosing *F. hepatica* infection in horses, cattle, and sheep. Although diagnostic sensitivities were above 85% for both ruminant species, the highest achieved value for horses was 28% (Palmer *et al.*, 2014). Thus, this assay is unlikely to become useful for horses without further modification and optimization.

Molecular diagnosis

Molecular techniques have shown great potential for diagnostic purposes, but very few have progressed to routine usage. However, progress in the development of PCR instrumentation and other platforms for DNA amplification suggest that these methods will become cheaper and more user-friendly in the near future. Accordingly, some of these pending advances are discussed herein.

The diagnostic potential of gene sequences encoding ribosomes has been reported extensively (Campbell, Gasser, and Chilton, 1995; Hung *et al.*, 1999) and led to several rDNA-based PCR assays for detecting important equine parasites. For example, a PCR assay has been developed for the detection of *Anoplocephala perfoliata* DNA in fecal samples (Drögemüller *et al.*, 2004). In a field study, however, this assay performed only slightly better than detection of eggs with the modified McMaster technique (Traversa *et al.*, 2008). Similarly, a multiplex PCR assay was developed to simultaneously detect DNA from all three anoplocephalid cestodes of horses with a detection limit of 50 eggs per sample (Bohorquez *et al.*, 2015). Again, the diagnostic sensitivity may need improvement before this assay can generate useful results in the field.

A PCR-ELISA for identifying six species of cyathostomins has proven reliable and applicable for detecting the presence of these species in fecal samples (Hodgkinson *et al.*, 2005). Similarly, a reverse line blot assay capable of detecting 21 species of cyathostomins and all three species of *Strongylus* has been developed and validated (Traversa *et al.*, 2007; Cwiklinski *et al.*, 2012). Both of these assays offer a qualitative test result (presence or absence of the parasite), whereas they provide no quantitative information about the abundance of the parasite species in question. A real-time PCR assay has been applied for the detection and semi-quantification of *Strongylus vulgaris* DNA in fecal samples (Nielsen *et al.*, 2008).

Ultrasonography

Given the lack of correlation between *Parascaris* spp. egg counts and worm burdens, an ultrasound technique was developed for transabdominally evaluating the small intestine for the presence of ascarid specimens in foals and assigning a semi-quantitative score for their abundance (Nielsen *et al.*, 2016). Examinations were performed with a portable ultrasound device using a 2.8 MHz convex probe and

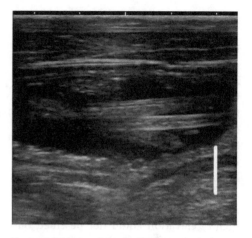

Figure 9.14 Transabdominal ultrasonographic image from a foal infected with *Parascaris* spp. present in the small intestine. Size bar = 1 cm.

foals were scanned at three locations along the ventral midline. Ascarids appear white and echogenic on the screen and the cuticle has a characteristic appearance of double, parallel lines in longitudinal section (Figure 9.14). An ascarid abundance score (1 to 4) and an ultrasonography quality score (A–F) were assigned. The majority of images (81%) were of acceptable quality (A–C) and the ascarid abundance score correlated statistically with intestinal worm counts. This procedure can be performed in about five minutes with little or no need for sedation. Furthermore, clipping is unnecessary during the summer months and soaking the ventral abdominal wall with ethanol or isopropyl alcohol is sufficient to facilitate images of good diagnostic quality.

Future diagnostics

Prepatent diagnosis of encysted cyathostomins

Several recent diagnostic developments show distinct promise and might become available in the relatively near future.

As mentioned in Chapter 2, encysted mucosal larvae are recognized as the main pathogenic stages of the cyathostomin life cycle, but coprologic methods cannot detect their presence. British scientists have isolated two antigens from encysted cyathostomins that offer potential for detecting prepatent worm burdens. Positive correlations have been reported between antibody titers and encysted worm burdens (Dowdall *et al.*, 2003). Molecular investigations have further identified and characterized the protein component of one antigen that did not cross-react with luminal stages or with other helminth species (McWilliam *et al.*, 2010; Mitchell *et al.*, 2016). This body of work shows great promise, but additional studies are required before a diagnostic assay can be made available. Given the fact that all horses harbor encysted cyathostomins, it is important that such an assay be at least semi-quantitative, differentiating between low, medium, and high numbers of encysted larvae.

Tapeworm copro-antigen ELISA

Copro-antigen ELISAs have shown some promise for detecting a number of helminth parasites. The basic premise is that antigens released by worms into the ingesta may be distributed more evenly than the eggs, which tend to occur in clusters. A copro-antigen ELISA for diagnosing the equine tapeworm *Anoplocephala perfoliata* has been developed (Kania and Reinemeyer, 2005) and validated, with 74% sensitivity and 92% specificity (Skotarek, Colwell, and Goater, 2010). This method therefore has potential to be applied in the field.

Automated smartphone-based fecal egg counts

A novel, egg-counting technology is able to exploit the high-resolution cameras installed in most modern smartphones. Measured fecal samples are suspended, filtered, and stained with a fluorescent dye conjugated to a chitin-binding domain (Figure 9.15). This material stains the nematode eggs, which are captured on a fine-mesh filter. A digital image is taken of the stained egg preparation and an image analysis application is used to recognize and count eggs based on shape and size (Slusarewicz *et al.*, 2016). This technology does not require a laboratory microscope and the filtering, staining, and counting processes are all automated so operator-dependency is reduced to collecting

Figure 9.15 Equine ascarid (round) and strongyle (ovoid) eggs stained with fluorescein and visualized via diagnostic imaging. A smartphone/computer tablet application has been developed to automatically count eggs present in a sample based on shape and size. (*Source*: Photograph courtesy of Dr. Paul Slusarewicz).

and measuring the sample and making the initial suspension. Work with an iPhone-based prototype has illustrated that this technology had significantly higher precision than the McMaster technique (Scare *et al.*, 2017). In comparison with the more refined Mini-FLOTAC

technique, the automated technology had a similar precision, but lower accuracy. Furthermore, this procedure reliably identifies and differentiates strongyle from ascarid egg types (Slusarewicz *et al.*, 2016). Plans for commercialization of this technology are currently underway.

References

Abbott, J.B., Mellor, D.J., and Love, S. (2007) Assessment of serum protein electrophoresis for monitoring therapy of naturally acquired equine cyathostomin infections. *Vet. Parasitol.*, 147, 110–117.

Abbott, J.B., Mellor, D.J., Barrett, E.J., *et al.* (2008) Serological changes observed in horses infected with *Anoplocephala perfoliata* after treatment with praziquantel and natural reinfection. *Vet. Rec.*, 162, 50–53.

Andersen, U.V., Howe, D.K., Dangoudoubiyam, S., *et al.* (2013) rSvSXP: A *Strongylus vulgaris* antigen with potential for prepatent diagnosis. *Parasit. Vectors*, 6, 84.

Bailey, M., Kent, J., Martin, S.C., *et al.* (1984) Haematological and biochemical values in horses naturally infected with *Strongylus vulgaris*. *Vet. Rec.*, 115, 144–147.

Bain, S.A. and Kelly, J.D. (1977) Prevalence and pathogenicity of *Anoplocephala perfoliata* in a horse population in South Auckland. *N. Z. Vet. J.* 25, 27–28.

Barda, B.D., Rinaldi, L., Ianniello, D., *et al.* (2013) Mini-FLOTAC, an innovative direct diagnostic technique for intestinal parasitic infections: experience from the field. *PLoS Negl. Trop. Dis.*, 7, 8.

Becher, A., Mahling, M., Nielsen, M.K., and Pfister, K. (2010) Selective anthelmintic therapy of horses in the Federal States of Bavaria (Germany) and Salzburg (Austria): An investigation into strongyle egg shedding consistency. *Vet. Parasitol.*, 171, 116–122.

Bellaw, J.L. and Nielsen, M.K. (2015) Evaluation of Baermann apparatus sedimentation time on recovery of *Strongylus vulgaris* and *S. edentatus* third stage larvae from equine coprocultures. *Vet. Parasitol.*, 211, 99–101.

Bevilaqua, C.M.L., Rodrigues. M. de L., and Concordet, D. (1993) Identification of infective larvae of some common nematode strongylids of horses. *Rev. Med. Vet.* 144, 989–995.

Bohorquez, A., Meana, A., and Luzon, M. (2012) Differential diagnosis of equine cestodosis based on E/S and somatic *Anoplocephala perfoliata* and *Anoplocephala magna* antigens. *Vet. Parasitol.*, 190, 87–94.

Bohorquez, A., Meana, A., Pato, N.F., and Luzon, M. (2014) Coprologically diagnosing *Anoplocephala perfoliata* in the presence of *A. magna*. *Vet. Parasitol.*, 204, 396–401.

Bohorquez, A., Luzon, M., Hernandez, R.M., and Meana, A. (2015) New multiplex PCR method for the simultaneous diagnosis of the three known species of equine tapeworm. *Vet. Parasitol.*, 207, 56–63.

Bracken, M.K., Wøhlk, C.B.M., Petersen, S.L., and Nielsen, M.K. (2012) Evaluation of conventional PCR for detection of *Strongylus vulgaris* on horse farms. *Vet. Parasitol.*, 184, 387–391.

Campbell, A.J., Gasser, R.B., and Chilton, N.B. (1995) Differences in a ribosomal DNA sequence of *Strongylus* species allows identification of single eggs. *Int. J. Parasitol.*, 25, 359–365.

Carstensen, H., Larsen, L., Ritz, C., and Nielsen, M.K. (2013) Daily variability of strongyle fecal egg counts in horses. *J. Equine Vet. Sci.*, 33, 161–164.

Cox, D.D. and Todd, A.C. (1962) Survey of gastrointestinal parasitism in Wisconsin dairy cattle. *J. Am. Vet. Med. Assoc.*, 141, 706–709.

Cringoli, G., Rinaldi, L., Maurelli, M.P., and Utzinger, J. (2010) FLOTAC: new multivalent techniques for qualitative and quantitative copromicroscopic diagnosis of parasites in animals and humans. *Nat. Protoc.*, 5, 503–515.

Cwiklinski, K., Kooyman, F.N.J., Van Doorn, D.C.K., *et al.* (2012) New insights into sequence variation in the IGS region of 21 cyathostomin species and the implication for molecular identification. *J. Parasitol.*, 1–11.

Dowdall, S.M., Proudman, C.J., Love, S., *et al.* (2003) Purification and analyses of the specificity of two putative diagnostic antigens for larval cyathostomin infection in horses. *Res. Vet Sci.*, 75, 223–229.

Drögemüller, M., Beelitz, P., Pfister, K., *et al.* (2004) Amplification of ribosomal DNA of Anoplocephalidae: *Anoplocephala perfoliata* diagnosis by PCR as a possible alternative to coprological methods. *Vet. Parasitol.*, 124, 205–215.

Duncan, J.L. (1974) Field studies on the epidemiology of mixed strongyle infections in the horse. *Vet. Rec.*, 94, 337–345.

Elsener, J. and Villeneuve, A. (2011) Does examination of fecal samples 24 hours after cestocide treatment increase the sensitivity of *Anoplocephala* spp. detection in naturally infected horses? *Can. Vet. J.*, 52, 158–161.

Gordon, H.M. and Whitlock, H.V. (1939) A new technique for counting nematode eggs in sheep faeces. *J. Counc. Scient. Ind. Res.*, 12, 50–52.

Greatorex, J.C. (1977) Diagnosis and treatment of "verminous aneurysm" formation in the horse. *Vet. Rec.*, 101, 184–187.

Hodgkinson, J.E., Freeman, K.L., Lichtenfels, J.R., *et al.* (2005) Identification of strongyle eggs from anthelmintic-treated horses using a PCR-ELISA based on intergenic DNA sequences. *Parasitol. Res.*, 95, 287–292.

Hung, G.-C., Gasser, R.B., Beveridge, I., and Chilton, N.B. (1999) Species-specific amplification by PCR of ribosomal DNA from some equine strongyles. *Parasitol.*, 119, 69–80.

Kania, S.A. and Reinemeyer, C.R. (2005) *Anoplocephala perfoliata* coproantigen detection: A preliminary study. *Vet. Parasitol.*, 127, 115–119.

Kaplan, R.M. and Nielsen, M.K. (2010) An evidence-based approach to equine parasite control: It ain't the 60s anymore. *Equine Vet. Educ.*, 22, 306–316.

Kent, J.E. (1987) Specific serum protein changes associated with primary and secondary *Strongylus vulgaris* infections in pony yearlings. *Equine Vet. J.*, 19, 133–137.

Kent, J.E. and Blackmore, D.J. (1985) Measurement of IgG in equine blood by immunoturbidimetry and latex agglutination. *Equine Vet. J.*, 17, 125–129.

Kjær, L.N., Lungholt, M.M., Nielsen, M.K., *et al.* (2007) Interpretation of serum antibody response to *Anoplocephala perfoliata* in relation to parasite burden and faecal egg count. *Equine Vet. J.*, 39, 529–533.

Klei, T.R. (1986) Laboratory diagnosis. *Vet. Clin. N. Am. Equine*, 2, 381–393.

Klei, T.R., Chapman, M.R., Torbert, B.J., and McClure, J.R. (1983) Antibody responses of ponies to initial and challenge infections of *Strongylus vulgaris*. *Vet. Parasitol.*, 12, 187–198.

Klei, T.R., Torbert, B., Chapman, M.R., and Foil, L.D. (1984) Prevalence of *Onchocerca cervicalis* in ponies. *J. Parasitol.*, 66, 859–861.

Kornas, S., Gawor, J., Cabaret, J., *et al.* (2009) Morphometric identification of equid cyathostome (Nematoda: Cyathostominae) infective larvae. *Vet. Parasitol.*, 162, 290–294.

Lester, H.E. and Matthews, J.B. (2014) Faecal worm egg count analysis for targeting anthelmintic treatment in horses: Points to consider. *Equine Vet. J.*, 46, 139–145.

Lester, H.E., Spanton, J., Stratford, C.H., et al. (2013) Anthelmintic efficacy against cyathostomins in horses in Southern England. *Vet. Parasitol.*, 197, 189–196.

Lightbody, K.L., Davis, P.J., and Austin, C.J. (2016) Validation of a novel saliva-based ELISA test for diagnosing tapeworm burden in horses. *Vet. Clin. Path.*, 45, 335–346.

McWilliam, H.E.G., Nisbet, A.J., Dowdall, S.M.J., et al. (2010) Identification and characterisation of an immunodiagnostic marker for cyathostomin developing stage larvae. *Int. J. Parasitol.*, 40, 265–275.

Mitchell, M.C., Tzelos, T., Handel, I., et al. (2016) Development of a recombinant protein-based ELISA for diagnosis of larval cyathostomin infection. *Parasitology*, 143, 1055–1066.

Nelis, H., Geurden, T.E., Charlier, J., et al. (2009) Development of a serum antibody elisa to detect *Fasciola hepatica* infections in horses. World Association for the Advancement of Veterinary Parasitology, Calgary, Canada, August 9–13, 2009, p. 185.

Nielsen, M.K. (2016) Equine tapeworm infections – disease, diagnosis, and control. *Equine Vet. Educ.*, 28, 388–395.

Nielsen, M.K., Haaning, N., and Olsen, S.N. (2006) Strongyle egg shedding consistency in horses on farms using selective therapy in Denmark. *Vet. Parasitol.*, 135, 333–335.

Nielsen, M.K., Peterson, D.S., Monrad, J., et al. (2008) Detection and semi-quantification of *Strongylus vulgaris* DNA in equine faeces by real-time PCR. *Int. J. Parasitol.*, 38, 443–453.

Nielsen, M.K., Vidyashankar, A., Andersen, U.V., et al. (2010a) Effects of fecal collection and storage factors on strongylid egg counts in horses. *Vet. Parasitol.*, 167, 55–61.

Nielsen, M.K., Baptiste, K.E., Tolliver, S.C., et al. (2010b) Analysis of multiyear studies in horses in Kentucky to ascertain whether counts of eggs and larvae per gram of feces are reliable indicators of numbers of strongyles and ascarids present. *Vet. Parasitol.*, 174, 77–84.

Nielsen, M.K., Vidyashankar, A.N., Bellaw, J., et al. (2014) Serum *Strongylus vulgaris*-specific antibody responses to anthelmintic treatment in naturally infected horses. *Parasitol. Res.*, 114, 445–451.

Nielsen, M.K., Scare, J.A., Gravatte, H.S., et al. (2015) Changes in serum *Strongylus vulgaris*-specific antibody concentrations in response to anthelmintic treatment of experimentally infected foals. *Front. Vet. Sci.*, 2, 17.

Nielsen, M.K., Donoghue, E.M., Stephens, M.L., et al. (2016) An ultrasonographic scoring method for transabdominal monitoring of ascarid burdens in foals. *Equine Vet. J.*, 48, 380–386.

Noel, M.L., Scare, J.A., Bellaw, J.L., and Nielsen, M.K. (2017) Accuracy and precision of Mini-FLOTAC and McMaster techniques for determining equine strongyle egg counts. *J. Equine Vet. Sci.* 48, 182–187.

Norris, J.K., Steuer, A., Scare, J.A., et al. (2017) The propensity of density: determining specific gravity of equine parasite eggs. *American Association for Veterinary Parasitologists Conference*, Indianapolis, Indiana, July 22–25, 2017.

Ogbourne, C.P. (1971) On the morphology, growth and identification of the pre-infective larvae of some horse strongylids. *Parasitol.*, 63, 455–472.

Olsen, S.N., Schumann, T., Pedersen, A., and Eriksen, L. (2003) Recovery of live immature cyathostome larvae from the faeces of horses by Baermann technique. *Vet. Parasitol.*, 116, 259–263.

Palmer, D.G., Lyon, J., Palmer, M.A., and Forshaw, D. (2014) Evaluation of a copro-antigen ELISA to detect *Fasciola hepatica* infection in sheep, cattle and horses. *Aust. Vet. J.*, 92, 357–361.

Patton, S., Mock, R.E., Drudge, J.H., and Morgan, D. (1978) Increase of immunoglobulin T concentration in ponies as a response to experimental infection with the nematode *Strongylus vulgaris. Am. J. Vet. Res.*, 39, 19–23.

Pearson, G.R., Davies, L.W., White, A.L., and O'Brien, J.K. (1993) Pathological lesions associated with *Anoplocephala perfoliata* at the ileo-caecal junction of horses. *Vet. Rec.*, 132, 179–182.

Poynter, D. (1954) Seasonal fluctuations in the number of strongyle eggs passed in horses. *Vet. Rec.*, 66, 74–78.

Presland, S.L., Morgan, E.R., and Coles, G.C. (2005) Counting nematode eggs in equine faecal samples. *Vet. Rec.*, 156, 208–210.

Proudman, C.J. and Edwards, G.B. (1992) Validation of a centrifugation/flotation technique for the diagnosis of equine cestodiasis. *Vet. Rec.*, 131, 71–72.

Rehbein, S., Lindner, T., Visser, M., and Winter, R. (2011) Evaluation of a double centrifugation technique for the detection of *Anoplocephala* eggs in horse faeces. *J. Helminthol.*, 85, 409–414.

Relf, V.E., Morgan, E.R., Hodgkinson, J.E., and Matthews, J.B. (2013) Helminth egg excretion with regard to age, gender and management practices on UK Thoroughbred studs. *Parasitology*, 140, 641–652.

Roepstorff, A. and Nansen, P. (1998) Epidemiology, diagnosis and control of helminth parasites of swine, in *FAO Animal Health Manual*, Rome, pp. 51–55.

Russell, A.F. (1948) The development of helminthiasis in Thoroughbred foals. *J. Comp. Path. Therap.*, 58, 107–127.

Sanada, Y., Senba, H., Mochizuki, R., *et al.* (2009) Evaluation of marked rise in fecal egg output after bithionol administration to horse and its application as a diagnostic marker for equine *Anoplocephala perfoliata* infection. *J. Med. Vet. Sci.*, 71, 617–620.

Scare, J.A., Slusarewicz, P., Noel, M.L., *et al.* (2017) Evaluation of accuracy and precision of a smartphone based automated parasite egg counting system in comparison to the McMaster and Mini-FLOTAC methods. *Vet. Parasitol.*, 247, 85–92.

Schultze, J.L., Bergfeld, W.A., and Wall, R.T. (1983) Serum protein electrophoresis as an aid in diagnosis of equine verminous arteritis. *Vet. Med. Sm. Anim. Clin.*, 78, 1279–1282.

Skotarek, S.L., Colwell, D.D., and Goater, C.P. (2010) Evaluation of diagnostic techniques for *Anoplocephala perfoliata* in horses from Alberta, Canada. *Vet. Parasitol.*, 172, 249–255.

Slusarewicz, P., Pagano, S., Mills, C., *et al.* (2016) Automated parasite fecal egg counting using fluorescence labeling, smartphone image capture and computational image analysis. *Int. J. Parasitol.*, 46, 485–493.

Stoll, N.R. (1923) Investigations on the control of hookworm disease. XV. An effective method of counting hookworm eggs in feces. *Am. J. Hyg.*, 3, 59–70.

Tomczuk, K., Kostro, K., Grzybek, M., *et al.* (2015) Seasonal changes of diagnostic potential in the detection of *Anoplocephala perfoliata* equine infections in the climate of Central Europe. *Parasitol. Res.*, 114, 767–772.

Traversa, D., Iorio, R., Klei, T.R., *et al.* (2007) New method for simultaneous species-specific identification of equine Strongyles (Nematoda, Strongylida) by reverse line blot hybridization. *J. Clin. Microbiol.*, 45, 2937–2942.

Traversa, D., Fichi, G., Campigli, M., *et al.* (2008) A comparison of coprological, serological and molecular methods for the diagnosis of horse infection with *Anoplocephala perfoliata* (Cestoda, Cyclophyllidea). *Vet. Parasitol.*, 152, 271–277.

Uhlinger, C. (1993) Uses of fecal egg count data in equine practice. *Comp. Cont. Educ. Vet. Pract.*, 15, 742–749.

Wallace, K.D., Selcer, B.A., Tyler, D.E., and Brown, J. (1989) Transrectal ultrasonography of the cranial mesenteric artery of the horse. *Am. J. Vet. Res.*, 50, 1699–1703.

Weiland, G., Hasslinger, M.A., Mezger, S., and Pollein, W. (1991) Possibilities and limits of immunodiagnosis of strongyle infections in horses. *Berl Munch. Tierarztl. Wochenschr.*, 104, 149–153.

10

Detection of Anthelmintic Resistance

Research with various parasites of other domestic mammals has resulted in the development and validation of molecular and *in vitro* assays for detection of anthelmintic resistance, but none of these has found application for horses. Perhaps the major difference between the strongyles of horses and the trichostrongylids of other livestock is the sheer number of cyathostomin species present in typical infections. It is not uncommon to find 15–20 different species infecting one horse, which undoubtedly contributes to the high variability observed in the test parameters evaluated.

The following section contains a short summary of technologies that are available for anthelmintic resistance detection, but not currently applicable to equids. The ability of benzimidazoles to kill developing larvae within a nematode egg has been exploited in an egg hatch inhibition test (EHT). Undeveloped eggs are isolated from fresh feces and incubated in varying concentrations of a soluble benzimidazole. The eggs of resistant worm strains are able to hatch at much higher BZ concentrations than those from known, susceptible isolates.

An EHT has recently been standardized for detection of benzimidazole resistance in ruminant nematodes (von Samson-Himmelstjerna *et al.*, 2009) and potentially could be used for horses. However, the egg hatch inhibition test has not been validated for horses. Regardless, the prevalence of BZ resistance in cyathostomin populations has approached ubiquity, so testing for its presence is irrelevant.

Larval development assays (LDA) have been validated for detection of anthelmintic resistance in ruminant trichostrongyles. The principle is to expose developing strongyle larvae to a range of drug concentrations and to evaluate efficacy by assessment of dose–response curves. Attempts to validate LDA for diagnosis of cyathostomin resistance were confounded by excessive variability in the data, resulting in marked overlap between susceptible and resistant strains, so the technique is not considered useful (Tandon and Kaplan, 2004; Lind *et al.*, 2005). Recent work with another *in vitro* method, the larval migration inhibition assay (LMIA), has shown promise for detection of ivermectin and moxidectin resistance in cyathostomins, and may become available in the future (Matthews *et al.*, 2012; McArthur *et al.*, 2015).

Molecular methods have been applied for detection of resistance, but these are hampered by the fact that relatively few genetic determinants have been identified. For benzimidazole resistance, single nucleotide polymorphisms (SNPs) that confer resistance have been identified and a Real-Time PCR assay has been developed for their detection (von Samson-Himmelstjerna *et al.*, 2003). However, given the high prevalence of benzimidazole resistance, its mere identification has

Handbook of Equine Parasite Control, Second Edition. Martin K. Nielsen and Craig R. Reinemeyer.
© 2018 John Wiley & Sons, Inc. Published 2018 by John Wiley & Sons, Inc.

little value. It would be more important to have molecular tools available for early detection of emerging resistance, such as to ivermectin and moxidectin, but these have not yet been developed. As mentioned in Chapter 8, the genetic mechanisms for anthelmintic resistance have yet to be unraveled and molecular methods for diagnosing resistance cannot be developed before this has been achieved.

Despite all these elegant laboratory exercises, only one technique constitutes a practical method for detecting anthelmintic resistance in horses, *i.e.*, the fecal egg-count reduction test (FECRT).

Fecal egg-count reduction test (FECRT)

An efficacious anthelmintic treatment will kill a large proportion of adult female worms, which are the sole source of parasite eggs passed in the feces. Thus, quantitative changes in egg numbers comprise a surrogate measure of adulticidal efficacy.

The underlying principle of the FECRT is extremely simple. The efficacy of an anthelmintic is evaluated and quantified by its ability to reduce fecal egg output after treatment in a group of horses. Fecal egg counts (FECpre) are performed just before (or at the time of) treatment and again 14 days after treatment (FECpost), and egg reduction for the tested group is calculated according to the formula:

$$\%FECR = \left(\frac{FECpre - FECpost}{FECpre} \right) \times 100$$

Although this seems very straightforward, livestock parasitologists are actively involved in esoteric discussions to develop detailed guidelines for further validation of FECRT to detect anthelmintic resistance

in horses. An expert committee has been formed under the World Association for the Advancement of Veterinary Parasitology (WAAVP), but new guidelines have yet to be published.

The following discussion presents recommendations that are based on the best information currently available.

Selection of egg-counting technique

Virtually any egg-counting technique can be employed for the FECRT, but a method with a detection limit of 25 or fewer eggs per gram is recommended. In cases of emerging resistance, post-treatment egg counts might be relatively low. If a technique with a higher detection limit were used, these few eggs may go undetected, and the FECR could be calculated (inaccurately) as 100%. As described in Chapter 9, the egg-counting techniques with lower limits of detection tend to be more time-consuming, so the advantages and disadvantages of any technique must be considered, depending on the circumstances. Regardless of choice, it is important to use the same technique consistently pre- and post-treatment.

The magnitude of the pre-treatment egg count is extremely important for the outcome of the FECRT. Let us consider an example in which a group of horses has a pre-treatment egg count of around 100 EPG, determined by an egg-counting technique with a detection limit of 25 EPG. If the drug being tested is 85% efficacious, the "true" observed post-treatment egg count should theoretically be around 15 eggs per gram for these horses. However, because 15 EPG is below the detection threshold of the quantitative test, the post-treatment result will most likely be reported (inaccurately) as 0 EPG for the majority of these horses, and efficacy will be calculated as close to 100%. If another group with pre-treatment egg counts of

Table 10.1 Suitability of horses with different pre-treatment egg count levels for inclusion in FECRT. Depending on the detection limit of the egg-counting technique used, some egg count levels may be too low for detecting reduced anthelmintic efficacy.

Detection limit	Pre-treatment egg count			
	0–200	200–500	500–1000	>1000
1 EPG	++	+++	+++	+++
10 EPG	+	++	+++	+++
25 EPG	-	+(+)	+++	+++
50 EPG	-	+	++	+++

+++: very suitable.
++: suitable.
+: avoid if possible.
-: do not use.

around 1000 EPG were treated with the same drug, they would be shedding around 150 EPG post-treatment. This number is well above the detection limit and the mean FECR will be substantially below 100% in this group. Therefore, FECRT efforts should preferentially use horses with moderate to high egg counts, especially when the egg-counting technique employed does not have a very low detection limit. Table 10.1 illustrates the relationship between egg-count ranges and FEC detection limits, and provides guidance for selecting horses and egg-count techniques for performing an FECRT. Precision (see Chapter 9 for a definition) is another important test quality to consider when choosing an appropriate egg-counting technique. A higher precision is preferred, as it reduces much of the random variability observed between repeated egg counts. Precision helps to discriminate between chance variation and true reduction. See Chapter 9 for examples of egg-counting techniques with high precision. The simplest advice for performing a good fecal egg count reduction test is to ensure that all tested horses have high pre-treatment FECs (>1000 EPG), as that would reduce the importance of the egg-counting technique employed. However, the majority of adult horses are low to moderate strongyle egg shedders, so this is much easier said than done.

Guidelines for diagnosing resistance

Anthelmintic resistance occurs at the parasite population level and variability among horses may be extreme. Therefore, FECRT should be estimated at the farm level by determining the FECR for a number of individual horses and then calculating the average FECR for the treated group. It is recommended that at least six horses, each with FEC ≥ 200 EPG, be included from each farm, if possible. Test results from groups of fewer than six horses should be interpreted with great caution, unless very high efficacy (>95%) or very low efficacy (<80%) is seen consistently among all the horses tested. Horses with pre-treatment FECs of "0" cannot be included in an FECRT.

In order to diagnose anthelmintic resistance, the expected efficacy of the drug being evaluated should be considered. Efficacies differ among various anthelmintics, but a reference standard can be found in the label claims for a product when it was first introduced to market. If efficacy data are not presented in the package insert, they can be found in Freedom of Information summaries posted on the web site of the relevant regulatory agency. As an example, pyrantel formulations were typically 95 to 100% effective at launch, whereas ivermectin and moxidectin had efficacies >99%. Therefore, suggested efficacy thresholds for indicating resistance depend on the drug class being evaluated as well as the number of horses tested. For a group of at least six horses, the following guidelines for minimal, acceptable efficacy should apply for equine strongyles:

Benzimidazoles: 95%
Pyrantel: 90%
Ivermectin: 95%
Moxidectin: 95%

The same cut-off values can probably be applied for *Parascaris* spp., although this assertion has not been confirmed by research. No available methods are capable of detecting anthelmintic resistance in equine tapeworms. The serum antibodies that are used for diagnosis remain elevated for months after treatment and methods for counting tapeworm eggs are insufficiently sensitive for post-treatment follow-up (see Chapter 9).

The requirement to measure two sets of FECs in a representative group of horses can be cumbersome or impractical, especially in foals and juveniles. In these situations, a pragmatic approach could be to evaluate only post-treatment samples. Although this will not provide an exact measure of efficacy, it will give some indication of treatment success because FECs should be low or negative after effective therapy. If post-treatment counts are higher than expected, the matter could be investigated further with a full FECRT.

Interpretation of FECRT

Although the mechanics of FECRT are relatively simple, interpretation of the results can be quite complicated.

Egg-count data are notoriously variable and it can be a challenge to take that variability into account when interpreting the results. As described in Chapter 9, individual egg counts vary in the range of ± 50%. In other words, each egg count should be viewed as one data point taken from a distribution with a certain mean and standard error. Unless we perform an infinite number of FECs from the same horse, we cannot know whether a certain egg count represents the true mean or if it is closer to the upper or lower extremes of the distribution. In Figure 10.1, egg count distributions from four different horses are presented.

One approach to establishing a more accurate estimate of the egg count for each horse is to perform two or three egg counts from the same fecal sample and calculate the mean value. Of course, this approach is laborious and therefore not likely to be performed in a busy veterinary practice. A more realistic approach is to make use of a technique known to have high precision, such as the FLOTAC or Mini-FLOTAC methods.

In addition to the variability among repeated egg counts for the same horse, an additional level of variability occurs between different horses on a farm. In the case of resistance, individual FECRT values will always fall within a wide range of values. Some horses may exhibit 100% efficacy, whereas others could show 70% or lower. This variability can be reduced by always including several horses in the FECRT and then calculating the mean value. A good rule of thumb is that efficacy should never be considered reduced unless it is observed in more than a single horse at a given farm. If all other tested horses had the expected level of egg-count reduction, the resulting group mean reduction could be due to administration error in that single horse.

In scientific studies, 95% confidence intervals of the mean are often calculated to establish a measure of the variability of the FECRT values (Coles *et al.*, 2006). If the

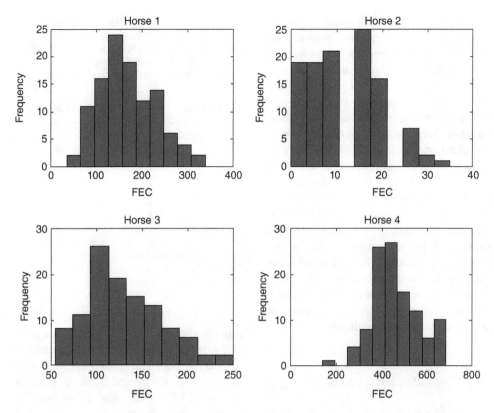

Figure 10.1 Variability in the egg count distributions of horses. The data in this figure represent 110 separate fecal egg counts (FECs) of the same horse, for four different horses. For each horse, five FECs were performed with each sample, and samples were collected approximately every 12 h over 11 days. Note the different magnitudes on the *x*-axis. (*Source*: Reprinted from Veterinary Parasitology, 185, Vidyashankar, A.N., Hanlon, B.M., and Kaplan, R.M., Statistical and biological considerations in evaluating drug efficacy in equine strongyle parasites using fecal egg-count data, pp. 45–57, Copyright (2012), with permission from Elsevier).

confidence intervals do not overlap with the predetermined cut-off values, this can be interpreted as a statistically supported loss of efficacy (*i.e.*, the variability exceeds that expected due to mere chance). It should be apparent that an estimate of anthelmintic efficacy will be more precise if more, rather than fewer, horses from a single farm are included in the FECRT.

If the farm average FECR falls below the cut-off values, anthelmintic resistance should be suspected. Given the variability described above, one should expect grey zones wherein the mean FECR is close to the cut-off values. In such cases, it is advisable to repeat the FECRT in the future before resistance is concluded.

Without calculating the confidence intervals, it is not possible to know when a certain result falls outside of the grey zone. However, as a rule of thumb, results within 5% of the cut-off should always be interpreted with great caution. If the sample size is smaller than six horses per farm, the grey zone should be expanded to 10%. With pyrantel, for example, the grey zone would be 85–90% and 80–90% if fewer than six horses are sampled. In general, FECRTs falling below the cut-off value should be reproducible. If an FECRT result cannot be reproduced, a conclusion of resistance is not warranted.

It is important to rule out other causes of decreased efficacy, such as intentional or unintentional under-dosing, partial loss of doses during administration, and reduced quality of drugs due to expiration or inappropriate storage. Establishment of accurate body weights is of paramount importance. If livestock scales are not available, the use of girth tapes is recommended. Because all current dewormers are administered orally, it is important to ensure that the entire dose is delivered and swallowed. Even though deworming is performed routinely and even rotely on many farms, it should be regarded as a significant therapeutic intervention. The short-term consequences matter whenever any portion of the intended dose ends up on the stall floor, and the long-term consequences are even more dire if careless dewormer administration is accepted by the farm's culture.

Egg reappearance periods

Egg reappearance periods (ERPs) were introduced in Chapter 9 and are widely used in equine parasitology. A working definition for ERP is "...the interval between an anthelmintic treatment and the time when parasite eggs can again be detected in the feces...." (See alternative definitions below.) The ERP was originally introduced as a tool for designing suppressive treatment regimens, but it now also has application as a surveillance tool for detecting evidence of declining efficacy in cyathostomin parasites. As described in Chapter 8, ERPs following ivermectin and moxidectin treatment reportedly have shortened considerably and this has been attributed to resistance by the luminal L_4 stage.

The range of ERPs for a particular anthelmintic may extend from a few weeks to the maximum interval identified when the drug was first approved for commercial distribution. Table 10.2 presents reports of cyathostomin ERPs for different anthelmintic drug classes in populations with no

Table 10.2 Cyathostomin egg reappearance periods (ERP) given in weeks post-treatment for different anthelmintic drugs in the absence of resistance. When anthelmintic resistance develops, ERPs are considerably shortened.

Anthelmintic	ERP (weeks)
Fenbendazole	6[a]
Pyrantel salts	5–6[b]
Ivermectin	9–13[c]
Moxidectin	16–22[d]

[a] McBeath *et al.*, 1978.
[b] Boersema *et al.*, 1995; 1996.
[c] Borgsteede *et al.*, 1993; Boersema *et al.*, 1996; Demeulenaere *et al.*, 1997.
[d] Jacobs *et al.*, 1995; DiPietro *et al.*, 1997; Demeulenaere *et al.*, 1997.

signs of anthelmintic resistance. As a general rule, ERPs in susceptible populations should be more than four weeks for fenbendazole and pyrantel, more than 9 weeks for ivermectin, and more than 16 weeks for moxidectin.

Definitions

Although the general concept of ERP is relatively straightforward, multiple definitions or criteria for measuring it have been proposed. Some authors have defined it as the week of the first positive egg count post-treatment (Dudeney, Campbell, and Coles, 2008, Lyons *et al.*, 2008). Others have used a fixed threshold for a mean egg count, such as 100 or 200 EPG (Boersema *et al.*, 1996; Mercier *et al.*, 2001). A third definition of ERP can be derived by performing FECRTs at weekly intervals post-treatment. The ERP is thereby defined as the interval when a calculated FECR falls below a predetermined cut-off value (Tarigo-Martinie, Wyatt, and Kaplan, 2001; Boersema *et al.*, 1995; von Samson-Himmelstjerna *et al.*, 2007).

The definition that relies on the first post-treatment positive count expects an initial FECR of 100% and fails to consider the variability introduced by the egg-counting technique. An anthelmintic need not reduce egg counts by 100% to be considered fully efficacious. In addition, using a fixed threshold, such as 100 or 200 EPG, can be biased by the herd structure in terms of low contaminator and high contaminator horses. Low contaminator horses will inadvertently take longer to reach a fixed threshold post-treatment than horses with higher pre-treatment egg counts. Therefore, an ERP definition based on contemporaneous FECR calculation represents a reasonable approach. The FECRT method considers the magnitude of pre-treatment egg counts and the designated cut-off values for the drug class used recently. Cut-off values should be tailored to the expected efficacy of the drug class being evaluated, and a conservative approach is to set ERP cut-offs approximately 10% lower than the resistance cut-offs presented previously in this chapter. Thus, the corresponding ERP cut-off values are:

Benzimidazoles: 85%
Pyrantel: 80%
Ivermectin: 85%
Moxidectin: 85%

As an example, the post-treatment interval during which the group mean FECR falls below 85% for a herd recently treated with moxidectin would define the ERP for that population, measured in weeks.

How to generate ERP information

When estimating ERP by the FECRT approach, standard considerations for the latter also apply (*e.g.*, number of horses sampled, pre-treatment FEC levels, sensitivity of the egg-counting technique, etc.). Egg reappearance periods are expressed, by convention, in units of "weeks post-treatment". Ideally, FECRTs should be performed weekly (after two weeks) until the cut-off value is reached, but that process is too laborious in a practice setting. A more pragmatic approach would be to target relevant time periods for the drug in question. For instance, the ERPs for pyrantel and fenbendazole are not expected to exceed four weeks, so ERP measurement would only be relevant at three weeks. Ivermectin and moxidectin have much longer ERPs, and it would be reasonable to begin screening at ~50% of the expected ERP. Thus, begin checking for evidence of ERP recovery at 3 to 4 weeks after treatment with ivermectin (which has an expected ERP of at least 9 weeks) and 4 to 6 weeks after moxidectin (with an expected ERP of at least 16 weeks).

It is important to emphasize that measuring ERP has no relevance once resistance has been detected because eggs first need to disappear before they can reappear. ERP surveillance, therefore, is currently more appropriate for tracking the efficacy of moxidectin and ivermectin against cyathostomins than for the other drug classes, in which resistance is more prevalent and operating at greater intensity.

References

Boersema, J.H., Borgsteede, F.H.M., Eysker, M., and Saedt, I. (1995) The reappearance of strongyle eggs in feces of horses treated with pyrantel embonate. *Vet. Quart.*, 17, 18–20.

Boersema, J.H., Eysker, M., Maas, J., and van der Aar, W.M. (1996) Comparison of the reappearance of strongyle eggs in foals, yearlings, and adult horses after treatment with ivermectin or pyrantel. *Vet. Quart.*, 18, 7–9.

Borgsteede, F.H.M., Boersma, J.H., Gaasenbeek, C.P.H., and Vanderburg, W.P.J. (1993) The reappearance of eggs in feces of horses after treatment with ivermectin. *Vet. Quart.*, 15, 24–26.

Coles, G.C., Jackson, F., Pomroy, W.E., *et al.* (2006) The detection of anthelmintic resistance in nematodes of veterinary importance. *Vet. Parasitol.*, 136, 167–185.

Demeulenaere, D., Vercruysse, J., Dorny, P., and Claerebout, E. (1997) Comparative studies of ivermectin and moxidectin in the control of naturally acquired cyathostome infections in horses. *Vet. Rec.*, 15, 383–386.

DiPietro, J.A., Hutchens, D.E., Lock, T.F., *et al.* (1997) Clinical trial of moxidectin oral gel in horses. *Vet. Parasitol.*, 72, 167–177.

Dudeney, A., Campbell, C., and Coles, G. (2008) Macrocyclic lactone resistance in cyathostomins. *Vet. Rec.*, 163, 163–164.

Jacobs, D.E., Hutchinson, M.J., Parker, L., and Gibbons, L.M. (1995) Equine cyathostome infection – suppression of faecal egg output with moxidectin. *Vet. Rec.*, 137, 545.

Lind, E.O., Uggla, A., Waller, P., and Hoglund, J. (2005) Larval development assay for detection of anthelmintic resistance in cyathostomins of Swedish horses. *Vet. Parasitol.*, 128, 261–269.

Lyons, E.T., Tolliver, S.C., Ionita, M., *et al.* (2008) Field studies indicating reduced activity of ivermectin on small strongyles in horses on a farm in Central Kentucky. *Parasitol. Res.*, 103, 209–215.

Matthews, J.B., McArthur, C., Robinson, A., and Jackson, F. (2012) The *in vitro* diagnosis of anthelmintic resistance in cyathostomins. *Vet. Parasitol.*, 185, 25–31.

McArthur, C.L., Handel, I.G., Robinson, A., *et al.* (2015) Development of the larval migration inhibition test for comparative analysis of ivermectin sensitivity in cyathostomin populations. *Vet. Parasitol.*, 212, 292–298.

McBeath, D.G., Best, J.M., Preston, N.K., and Duncan, J.L. (1978) Studies on the faecal egg output of horses after treatment with fenbendazole. *Equine Vet. J.*, 10, 5–8.

Mercier, P., Chick, B., Alves-Branco, F., and White, C.R. (2001) Comparative efficacy, persistent effect, and treatment intervals of anthelmintic pastes in naturally infected horses. *Vet. Parasitol.*, 99, 29–39.

Tandon, R. and Kaplan, R.M. (2004) Evaluation of a larval development assay (DrenchRite®) for the detection of anthelmintic resistance in cyathostomin nematodes of horses. *Vet. Parasitol.*, 121, 125–142.

Tarigo-Martinie, J.L., Wyatt, A.R., and Kaplan, R.M. (2001) Prevalence and clinical implications of anthelmintic resistance in cyathostomes of horses. *J. Am. Vet. Med. Assoc.*, 218, 1957–1960.

Vidyashankar, A.N., Hanlon, B.M., and Kaplan, R.M. (2012) Statistical and biological considerations in evaluating drug efficacy in equine strongyle parasites using fecal egg-count data, in *Veterinary Parasitology*, Elsevier, pp. 45–57.

von Samson-Himmelstjerna, G., Buschbaum, S., Wirtherle, N., *et al.* (2003) TaqMan minor groove binder real-time PCR analysis of beta-tubulin codon 200 polymorphism in small strongyles (Cyathostomin) indicates that the TAC allele is only moderately selected in benzimidazole-resistant populations. *Parasitology*, 127, 489–496.

von Samson-Himmelstjerna, G., Fritzen, B., Demeler, J., *et al.* (2007) Cases of reduced cyathostomin egg-reappearance period and failure of *Parascaris equorum* egg count reduction following ivermectin treatment as well as survey on pyrantel efficacy on German horse farms. *Vet. Parasitol.*, 144, 74–80.

von Samson-Himmelstjerna, G., Coles, G.C., Jackson, F., *et al.* (2009) Standardization of the egg hatch test for the detection of benzimidazole resistance in parasitic nematodes. *Parasitol. Res.*, 105, 825–834.

11

Evaluating Historical Information

Parasitism is a common differential diagnosis for various clinical conditions of
horses. However, the usual collection of
history-generating questions is often
inadequate for including or excluding
parasitism as a definitive diagnosis.
Clinicians are reminded that parasitism
embodies the classic epidemiologic tri-
angle of host, organism, and environment. Of these key factors, environment
is the most complicated because it incor-
porates climate, habitat (facilities), and
management interventions. Assessment
of the likelihood of parasitic disease
could be improved greatly if the anam-
nestic process were expanded to include
environmental factors that influence the
transmission of parasites.

Any number of approaches may be
implemented for collecting an adequate
parasitologic history for horses, and that
process is best left to the experience of
the practitioner. Regardless of personal
preferences, the process should include
information generated by asking the six
classic questions learned by every journalism student: Who? What? When?
Where? Why? How?

Who?

The "who" of our interrogatory process is
the equine host. The specific subject of
any history could be an individual horse,
or a discrete herd under specific management circumstances, or even an entire
farm comprised of multiple bands with
varying management systems.

The single host characteristic that has
the greatest impact on the distribution of
equine parasitism is age. However, host
age *per se* is usually just a surrogate parameter for other phenomena involved
in a host/parasite interaction. Thus,
Strongyloides westeri infections are seen
mostly in suckling foals and recent weanlings, not just because these animals are
young but because this organism is primarily transmitted vertically from the
dam to her offspring by the transmam-
mary route (see Chapter 1). The unique
age distributions of other parasitisms
within a population may actually reflect
the acquisition of protective immunity.
The prime example is *Parascaris* spp. burdens, which typically reach their peak at 4
to 5 months of age, after which they gradually decline. Doubtless, older horses also
ingest infective ascarid eggs on a continuous basis, but various immune processes
prevent those exposures from culminat-
ing in mature parasites. Historically, pinworms have also been uncommon in
mature horses, but this pattern may be
changing (Reinemeyer and Nielsen, 2014).

Host age can also help to prioritize differential diagnoses when it is compared to
the known prepatent periods of potential
parasitic pathogens. Thus, strongylid eggs

Handbook of Equine Parasite Control, Second Edition. Martin K. Nielsen and Craig R. Reinemeyer.
© 2018 John Wiley & Sons, Inc. Published 2018 by John Wiley & Sons, Inc.

observed in the feces of a 2 week old foal cannot possibly indicate the presence of adult worms in the foal's gut because the minimum prepatent period (PPP) for cyathostomins is around 5.5 weeks (see Chapter 1). Coprophagy is normal behavior in foals, but this ingestive practice may lead to false positive egg counts in this age group. In contrast, one validation study illustrated that the false-positive rate for *Parascaris* spp. egg counts in horses younger than 2 years of age was just 5% (Nielsen *et al.*, 2010). Thus, false positive fecal results are not a huge issue for this parasite, especially in an age group with a very high prevalence of infection. Similarly, strongyle eggs in the feces of a 4 month old foal denote a reproducing cyathostomin population, but those same eggs could not have been produced by large strongyles because the required PPP is greater than the host age.

Age also plays a significant role in the severity of damage inflicted by a parasitic infection. Adult horses are more resilient to parasitism than younger animals with less immunity, so the clinical effects tend to be much less severe in mature equids. Of course, this pattern can be modified by individual predispositions due to stress, immunosuppression, or concurrent disease.

At the extreme end of the age scale, geriatric horses are reported to have higher strongyle egg counts than mature horses (Adams *et al.*, 2015). While this is not necessarily associated with a risk of compromised health, geriatric horses may need more intensive parasite control than mature animals.

Sex of the animal is another host factor that may be an important variable for parasite susceptibility. Intact male sheep, goats, and cattle generally harbor significantly greater numbers of adult worms, have higher egg counts, and are more likely to suffer negative health consequences from a given type of parasite than intact females (Herd, Queen, and Majewski, 1992). Consistent with this pat-

tern, neutered males are often intermediate between the two sexes in their susceptibility to parasitism. A similar pattern has been observed in foals, wherein colts had significantly greater burdens of encysted cyathostomin larvae than fillies (Nielsen and Lyons, 2017). Interestingly, the opposite trend was observed with *Parascaris* spp. worm counts in a large cohort of foals; fillies had significantly greater intestinal burdens than colts (Fabiani, Lyons, and Nielsen, 2016). Clearly, the influence of host gender on parasite susceptibility needs to be studied more thoroughly in horses before any general rules can be formulated.

Although no breed predilections have been described for parasitisms of horses, minor differences exist between host species within the family Equidae. For example, donkeys and burros are the usual definitive hosts of the equine lungworm, *Dictyocaulus arnfieldi*, but this nematode does not mature or reproduce well in horses (*Equus caballus*). Similarly, but of no clinical significance, a few cyathostomin species are recovered exclusively from donkeys, but apparently do not infect horses grazing the same pastures (Tolliver, 2000).

Lastly, the question of "who" might even refer to an individual horse whenever a herd experiences new parasitic issues never encountered previously. In such cases, the clinician should investigate any new introductions to the herd and attempt to acquire as much information as possible about its origin and anthelmintic history, plus its relevant management since taking up residence on the farm.

What?

For purposes of this discussion, we designate the historical "what?" of parasitism as the various helminth species that can infect equids. The likelihood of a specific parasite being the cause of a clinical problem varies with its prevalence, pathogenicity, host

Table 11.1 Prevalence, pathogenicity, host interactions, and life cycle details influencing clinical parasitism in horses.

Parasite	Prevalence	Pathogenicity	Host Interactions	Life cycle detail
Cyathostomins	Ubiquitous	Typically not very pathogenic	Disease is rare except when mass larval emergence occurs	Acquired immunity may modulate disease and egg shedding, but not infection
Large strongyles	Currently absent or inconsequential in many herds	Can be severely pathogenic	Various clinical signs from colic to peritonitis	Immunity may modulate disease, but does not preclude infection
Parascaris spp.	Ubiquitous; occurs almost exclusively in juveniles	Varies from no effect to fatal consequences	Weight loss, diarrhea, poor growth, intestinal obstruction	Acquired immunity ultimately controls all ascarid infections
Oxyuris equi	Ubiquitous; more common in immature horses	Negligible pathogens	Anal pruritus	Adult horses presumably develop immunity
Strongyloides westeri	Low prevalence in many herds	Modest pathogen	Most infections are asymptomatic; can cause watery diarrhea	Ultimately controlled by acquired immunity
Gasterophilus spp.	Ubiquitous	Minimal	Egg-laying by adults is bothersome	Infections recur annually
Anoplocephala perfoliata	Ubiquitous in pastured horses	Varies from no effect to fatal consequences	Routine effects are unknown; serious consequences require surgery	No evidence of acquired immunity

interactions, and details of its life cycle. Those factors were presented in Chapters 1 and 2, but are summarized in Table 11.1 for the major internal parasites of horses.

When?

"When" may be the most important question in the collection and answering it requires detailed knowledge of parasite life cycles, epidemiology, and climatic conditions of the premise being investigated. The life cycles of most equine parasites are fairly protracted, which is an important point to impress upon horse clients. The bots they see passing in the feces during spring actually began as eggs on the haircoat many

months previously. Also, even the core, scripted features of a life cycle can be prolonged beyond recognition by the vagaries of environmental persistence and arrested development. Thus, a new foal may experience a *Parascaris* infection even though the farm has not sheltered other juveniles for a year or two, and individual horses can harbor egg-shedding cyathostomins despite several months of confinement and superior sanitation.

Strongyles and many other equine parasites are transmitted according to predictable, seasonal patterns (see Chapter 3). Knowledge of those patterns not only aids in predicting the seasons and circumstances of peak risk, but also helps to identify intervals when chemical control measures are unnecessary. Nearly every climate features some intervals when little parasite transmission occurs (see Chapter 3), and thus there is no need for treatment.

Time is an extremely important variable to consider when assessing the efficacy of control measures, and rigorous temporal guidelines for assessing FECR have been presented in this volume. As an example, deeming a dewormer ineffective because egg counts were moderately high at 6 weeks post-treatment is a false indictment in many cases (see Chapter 10). Temporal reconciliation of diagnostic results and historical information requires knowledge of the predictable declines in egg-count post-treatment, the expected duration of egg reappearance periods after effective therapy, and quantitative variations that would constitute evidence of anthelmintic resistance.

Where?

Nearly all parasitisms can be transmitted on pasture, but only some can cycle in confinement. For instance, the hardy eggs of ascarids and pinworms are very self-sufficient and might have less habitat preference. Strongyles prefer pasture habitats, but third stage larvae can be recovered from stall bedding (Love *et al.*, 2016), and doubtless some strongylid transmission occurs in confined horses. Tapeworms are transmitted exclusively on pasture, due to the essential role of free-living oribatid mites. However, one of the authors has observed cestode transmission in confined ruminants that were fed large bales of hay that had been stored outside. Soil mites apparently can invade hay bales stored in contact with the ground, and thus may be carried indoors to confined animals. Management sometimes confounds biology, and clinicians should always be on the lookout for exceptions to any rule.

"Where" is a very reasonable question whenever horses develop a parasitic issue

they have not experienced in the past. The simplest explanation for the appearance of an unfamiliar bug is that the hosts must have acquired it from a different environment. For example, investigation of lungworms as a diagnostic differential for pulmonary disease should include questions about historical exposure to venues with resident donkeys.

Although the examples are few in number, specific microhabitats have been identified as significant risk factors for certain parasitisms. Thus, damp sawdust bedding has been incriminated in clinical dermatitis ("frenzy") associated with *Strongyloides westeri* infection, and persistent wetlands are invariably present on pastures grazed by horses that acquire *Fasciola* infections. The udder of a foaling mare is yet another specific location from which a suckling foal could acquire parasitism in the form of infective *Parascaris* eggs.

Why and How?

The "why" and "how" of parasitism are similar questions that basically reiterate life cycle details and the modes of pathogenicity. However, numerous host and environmental variables become critically relevant when trying to explain why simple parasitism sometimes morphs into clinical disease. Constituent host factors have been addressed already in this chapter and in Chapter 4.

Environmental factors that have not yet been addressed include unique management features. We know that parasitic disease is a quantitative phenomenon, so one must consider any and all factors that could have resulted in a highly infective environment. The usual culprits include a high stocking rate on permanent pastures, particularly if grazed by young horses that tend to have higher egg counts than mature animals. The ill-advised practice of spreading uncomposted manure could also result in unusually high levels of infectivity.

Another contributing factor could be administration of an anthelmintic that failed to reduce contamination for some reason. Potential explanations for treatment failures include under-dosing and anthelmintic resistance. Other scenarios are more complicated, such as administering a non-larvicidal dewormer during a season when the majority of the cyathostomin population is in arrested development.

Other considerations

Although classic journalism questions help to define the science of parasite history-taking, the art includes other factors that are more difficult to characterize.

The significance of absence

The following conversation takes place in Conan Doyle's famous mystery story about the disappearance of a champion race horse (Silver Blaze):

> "Is there any point to which you would wish to draw my attention?"
> "To the curious incident of the dog in the night-time."
> "The dog did nothing in the night-time."
> "That was the curious incident," remarked Sherlock Holmes.

This literary episode demonstrates that valuable information can be deduced when something that should be present is inexplicably absent. For example, cyathostomins are ubiquitous in all horses except neonates, and even low contaminator adults are likely to be passing some eggs. Thus, the total absence of strongyle eggs in fecal samples from an entire herd is an unnatural situation, and the most likely explanations are recent, effective anthelmintic treatment or laboratory error. Therefore, when treatment history is unavailable but diagnostic results include a predominance of "0" egg counts, recent deworming is a feasible explanation.

On a related matter, the absence of eggs doesn't rule out the presence of worms, or even of parasitic disease (see Chapter 9). Indeed, this circumstance is commonplace in tapeworm infections, for which the sensitivity of many fecal diagnostic tests is very low (Chapter 9). Similarly, foals in the 0 to 3 month old range can harbour occult ascarid infections, and any horse may experience verminous arteritis, because both circumstances involve larval nematodes that are migrating systemically. Larvae are simply not mature enough to begin laying eggs. The absence of a patent infection today is no guarantee of freedom from serious parasitic problems in a month or so (*e.g.*, *Parascaris*), or even concurrently (larval cyathostominosis).

Don't over-interpret

It is important to recognize that most of the equine parasites listed in Table 11.1 are highly prevalent, so finding diagnostic evidence of their presence in a horse has few clinical implications. For instance, the passage of strongyle eggs by horses is extremely common, so finding eggs in the feces of a horse with colic symptoms should not be interpreted as comprising a causal relationship. Similarly, vague or unexplained clinical signs should not be attributed to *Anoplocephala* infection just because an ELISA from that horse revealed tapeworm-specific antibodies. The mere presence of a parasite is insufficient evidence to confirm disease, and certainly doesn't justify treatment. However, we appreciate that empirical treatment of an individual horse is a reasonable approach when definitive diagnosis is either impractical or expensive. Empirical treatment of entire herds, however, is a very bad idea.

A clinical diagnosis of parasitic disease can only be reached by considering all the information gathered during the interview process, described previously.

Diagnoses are typically reached by pattern recognition and an inclusion/exclusion approach. In the example of a horse with acute onset of watery diarrhea, it would be relevant to consider its age (is it younger than 5 years old?), the time of year (is it winter or early spring?), and previous deworming regimen (was it recently dewormed with a non-larvicidal anthelmintic?). Furthermore, it would be relevant to evaluate white blood cell counts and plasma protein concentrations. If the answer to the majority of these questions is "yes" and the horse has neutrophilia and hypoproteinemia, we have a pattern that strongly suggests larval cyathostominosis. Ultrasonography may help to visualize edematous large intestinal walls, but fecal egg counts or the Baermann procedure for larval recovery are not going to provide useful information. Like all infectious agents, however, parasites can contribute to any disease complex without being the primary cause.

Gastrointestinal helminth parasites of livestock exist as populations distributed within a herd of animals, yet parasitic diseases infrequently occur in epidemic form. The parasitologic picture of a herd equals the sum of the situations in multiple, individual horses, so a single animal may not accurately represent the typical situation within a host population. The corollary of this observation is that a single case of clinical disease is no indication that the remainder of the herd is destined to develop the same signs. However, clinical disease in even one individual indicates that something is obviously suboptimal, which is an excellent reason to review the parasite management practices of the farm.

Lastly, it should be emphasized yet again that anthelmintic efficacy can only be evaluated in a population and that FECRT should not be attempted with a single horse (see Chapter 10).

References

Adams, A.A., Betancourt, A., Barker, V.D., *et al.* (2015) Comparison of the immunologic response to anthelmintic treatment in old versus middle-aged horses. *J. Equine Vet. Sci.*, 35, 873–881.

Fabiani, J.V., Lyons, E.T., and Nielsen, M.K. (2016) Dynamics of *Parascaris* and *Strongylus* spp. parasites in untreated juvenile horses. *Vet. Parasitol.*, 30, 62–66.

Herd, R.P., Queen, W.G., and Majewski, G.A. (1992) Sex-related susceptibility of bulls to gastrointestinal parasites. *Vet. Parasitol.*, 44, 119–125.

Love, S., Burden, F.A., McGirr, E.C., *et al.* (2016) Equine Cyathostominae can develop to infective third-stage larvae on straw bedding. *Parasite Vector*, 9, 478.

Nielsen, M.K. and Lyons, E.T. (2017) Encysted cyathostomin larvae in foals – progression of stages and the effect of seasonality. *Vet. Parasitol.*, 236, 108–112.

Nielsen, M.K., Baptiste, K.E., Tolliver, S.C., *et al.* (2010) Analysis of multiyear studies in horses in Kentucky to ascertain whether counts of eggs and larvae per gram of feces are reliable indicators of numbers of strongyles and ascarids present. *Vet. Parasitol.*, 174, 77–84.

Reinemeyer, C.R. and Nielsen, M.K. (2014) Review of the biology and control of *Oxyuris equi. Equine Vet. Educ.*, 26, 584–591.

Tolliver, S.C. (2000) A practical method of identification of the North American cyathostomes (small Strongyles) in equids in Kentucky. Kentucky Agricultural Experiment Station, University of Kentucky, Lexington, KY.

12

Synopsis of Evidence-Based Parasite Control

When veterinary practitioners and horse owners turn to parasitologists for advice and guidance, the experience commonly results in annoyance, frustration, or wholesale rejection of any "new-fangled" recommendations. Those involved with the practical aspects of equine management typically seek simple and straightforward advice, and parasite control in horses has long been just that – a one-size-fits-all generic recipe in which the only variables are a drug and the calendar. Unfortunately, effective, sustainable, evidence-based parasite control is more complicated than most pragmatists suspect, and this book has attempted to explain why.

It is a very interesting exercise to ask clients, "Why do you deworm your horses?" Typical responses will touch on health maintenance, prevention of morbidity and mortality, and optimizing performance. However, in addition, other, baseless reasons such as "tradition" and "it's a mandatory management procedure" always emerge if one continues to press.

The core of evidence-based parasite control (EBPC) is based on reasons that are supported by scientific facts. Thus, first and foremost, it is of paramount importance to define the reasons for, or the goals of, a parasite control program. Whether or not clients can verbalize what they are striving for, veterinarians must translate their objectives into EBPC terms.

Currently, the goals for equine parasite control can be defined as follows:

- To minimize the risk of parasitic disease.
- To reduce infection pressure.
- To maintain and prolong the efficacy of existing anthelmintics.

Goals for parasite control have been revised during past decades and they are likely to change again in the future as new knowledge emerges and new tools are developed. Inherent to pursuing these goals is the recognition of certain basic facts: (1) parasitism is a natural state of livestock and cannot be eradicated; (2) parasitic disease, or at least the negative impacts on health, cannot be avoided entirely, regardless of the control regimen implemented; and (3) control measures must be tailored to the conditions on each farm.

Considering the evidence

It should be unnecessary to mention that ignoring the evidence is the most hazardous approach of all. Nonetheless, this happens routinely in the realm of equine parasite control. A calendar-based anthelmintic treatment regimen, performed without surveillance of efficacy or a consideration of which parasites are present, systematically ignores most of the scientific evidence presented in this book.

Handbook of Equine Parasite Control, Second Edition. Martin K. Nielsen and Craig R. Reinemeyer.
© 2018 John Wiley & Sons, Inc. Published 2018 by John Wiley & Sons, Inc.

It is impossible to make useful recommendations without detailed information about each farm and its control history. However, it is possible to present the key elements of a parasite control strategy, and those will serve as the scaffold on which a customized program can be assembled. In the following, we present several key elements that should exist in any parasite control program.

Measuring drug efficacy

As discussed in Chapter 9, the single most important reason for performing egg counts is to measure treatment efficacy by means of fecal egg count reduction testing (FECRT). The starting point for every farm is to evaluate the efficacy of what they are currently doing. Treatment with no assurance of efficacy creates a false sense of security, and populations of resistant worms can accumulate within the horses despite the labor and expense of misguided control efforts. As a rule of thumb, FECRTs should be performed on a yearly basis with each class of anthelmintic that was still effective last year. Details are presented in Chapter 10.

Basic treatment foundation

Parasite control programs are not unlike tract houses in any suburb. They differ in their details, but they all rest on a fairly similar foundation. In regard to horses, the foundation would be some control measure that is applied equally to all horses on a farm. Such measures are intended to minimize the prevalence of pathogenic parasites and to limit the numbers acquired by susceptible foals and juvenile horses.

Data from Denmark, where anthelmintic treatments are restricted to prescription-only use, suggest that large strongyle infections recrudesce if some horses on a farm are left completely untreated (Chapter 7). However, it does not require many anthelmintic treatments to suppress large strongyles. Given the long prepatent periods of *Strongylus* spp., one or two larvicidal treatments (ivermectin or moxidectin) within the annual cycle should reduce transmission considerably. Neither pyrantel nor a single dose of a benzimidazole will kill migrating larvae, so these are inappropriate for this purpose. The best time to apply such a treatment is toward the end of the grazing season. This will usually coincide with autumn in temperate climates, or during spring in warmer climates. At a maximum, treatments could be administered twice annually, at regular, 6 month intervals.

As outlined in Chapter 2, the risk of parasitic disease is low in well-managed horses, but it is clear from the literature that the risk of developing disease is greater in young horses. *Parascaris* spp. are primarily a threat to foals and yearlings, and horses under the age of five years are at greater risk of developing larval cyathostominosis. In addition, young horses are more likely to be high strongyle egg shedders. These facts suggest that young horses require more intensive treatment than adults. The treatment needs of this age group depend on numerous factors, and should be customized for the management of each farm. Regardless, a few general rules can be followed to design control strategies for breeding farms.

Foals

As a rough guideline, most foals should have the benefit of approximately four to five anthelmintic treatments during their first 15 months of life. A greater number would require firm justification based on high infection pressure or clinical problems in the herd. Fewer than four treatments would be considered inadequate in most cases.

The major helminth pathogen in foals younger than six months of age is *Parascaris* spp. Ideally, ascaricidal treatments should be timed as soon as possible after achievement of patency, but, without frequent monitoring, it is impossible to determine such optimal timing. Therefore, the first anthelmintic treatment of foals is recommended around the age of 2.5 to 3 months. Considering the increased risk of impactions from anthelmintics with a neuromuscular mode of action (see Chapter 7), benzimidazoles may be the best drug choice at this time. A second deworming treatment should be targeted around or just before the time of weaning. This is a stressful period for the foal and large parasite burdens would just compound the situation. The main parasitic threat at this time is still likely to be *Parascaris* spp., but strongyle parasites may start to play a role as well. Therefore, pre-weaning fecal egg counts yield useful information about the presence of ascarids and strongyles, and help guide the veterinarian in anthelmintic selection. While benzimidazoles would still be chosen for ascarid control, they are unlikely to also be effective against cyathostomins, so other drug classes need to be considered as well. A third treatment for yearlings should be implemented at around 8–10 months of age and should include consideration of tapeworm control. Drug selection at this time will depend on the results of yearly FECRTs performed on the farm, but should be directed primarily at strongyles. Egg counts may reveal low level ascarid infections in some individuals, and those should be treated accordingly. After foals become yearlings, parasite management should mirror the rhythm of adult horses, with treatments in the spring and early autumn. In areas with defined grazing seasons, a third treatment should be considered about midway through the grazing season and in areas where grazing seasons extend into November, a fourth treatment should be considered late in the

year. Yearlings are considerably more susceptible to parasitic infection than older horses and yearlings could easily acquire large parasite burdens if left untreated for longer periods during a grazing season of 5 to 9 months in duration.

Young horses

Treatment regimens will vary among farms for horses between one and approximately four years of age. Most programs resemble a compromise between a program appropriate for yearlings and one recommended for adult horses. Many farms would be justified to administer three treatments to this age group within an annual cycle. The three treatments could be scheduled before, midway, and toward the end of the grazing season. Cyathostomin larvicidal treatments using moxidectin or fenbendazole (where efficacious) might be considered for the final annual treatment in this age group. Again, it is important to consider tapeworm control by including cestocidal anthelmintics at least once during the grazing season.

Other considerations

Control efforts against the tapeworm *Anoplocephala perfoliata* should be considered in most regions. Current diagnostic tools for tapeworm detection have clear limitations (see Chapter 9), so routine screening for this parasite in entire herds is rarely feasible. However, testing a representative sample of the horses for tapeworm antibodies will at least reflect the level of tapeworm exposure and suggest the presence of infection within the herd. A pragmatic approach could combine tapeworm treatment with the foundation measures. Combination anthelmintics (praziquantel plus ivermectin or moxidectin) are ideal for this use. The best timing for cestode treatment is near the end of the grazing season, which is identical to the recommended scheduling for large strongyle larvicidal measures. If tapeworm antibodies indicate high levels of exposure, an additional treatment within the annual cycle could be considered.

Incidental diagnoses may indicate that some herds would benefit from additional treatments to control non-alimentary parasitisms, such as cutaneous habronemiasis or onchocerciasis.

Farm strategies, adult horses

As outlined in Chapter 7, fecal egg counts can be used systematically to identify adult horses with consistently low, moderate, or high levels of strongyle egg shedding. Currently, there are no incentives for treatment of low egg shedders beyond the foundation treatments suggested previously. Two annual treatments should suffice for most low and moderate shedders, depending on climate and infection pressure. High egg shedders will require additional treatments (Chapter 7). However, applying such treatments routinely to all horses in the herd has no biological or medical justification. Treating adult horses during the off-season is similarly unjustified if parasites were managed adequately during the active transmission season.

What is expected in the future?

Detailed advice has a limited shelf life because new knowledge will always force us to modify our recommendations in the future. The only reasonable accommodation is to make the best use of the knowledge presently at hand and to remain open to new information and be willing to change our parasite management accordingly. Experience has shown us how difficult this can be, and the present book is just the most recent installment in a series of efforts to equip veterinarians and their clients with the tools and knowledge to make such changes.

Although prediction is impossible, we can identify some potential research developments that would convince us to adjust our recommendations. A few examples are presented in the following.

Improved diagnostic tools?

More accurate diagnostic tools would enable us to develop and refine better strategies. For example, diagnostic tests capable of quantifying burdens of non-patent infections would be a superior indicator of the risk of potential parasitic disease in comparison to our current egg counts and larval cultures. Such tests would be extremely valuable for encysted cyathostomin larvae or prepatent *Parascaris* infections. Similarly, an accurate and quantitative method for estimating tapeworm burdens would be seminal for finally developing evidence-based control strategies for *Anoplocephala*. As outlined in Chapter 9, some recent developments in these fields have been promising.

Last but not least, less laborious tests for detection of anthelmintic resistance would greatly simplify the present dual-sample procedures and could remove much of the uncertainty with FECR calculations that fall in the "gray area" (see Chapter 10). The automated egg counting technology described in Chapter 9 may represent a less laborious and more reliable way to generate FECR data. Similarly, we cannot detect anthelmintic resistance in tapeworms or pinworms at this time.

Risk of disease?

Very few epidemiologic studies have evaluated the risk of disease associated with various parasite burdens or different anthelmintic treatment regimens. Such studies are essential and would likely lead to adjustments in our recommendations. The emerging diagnostic tools for detecting migrating or encysted parasite larvae, as mentioned previously, would be extremely useful for conducting such studies in the future.

Changes of biology?

In addition to selecting for anthelmintic resistance, chemically based management programs have probably also selected for changes in other biological traits of the target populations. Such changes may include shorter prepatent periods or entire life cycles, adaptation to a different host age spectrum, and changes in pathogenic potential. The history of parasitology abounds with examples of parasites that were initially considered harmless to their hosts, but subsequently were found to be of potential clinical importance. For horses, cyathostomins and tapeworms comprise such examples. We must also remember that the historical standards of "harm" were tantamount to clinical disease. The tenets of modern production agriculture have shown repeatedly that pathogenic organisms need not cause obvious harm to result in economic loss, or to compromise host health through immunosuppression and other non-specific mechanisms.

Further development of anthelmintic resistance?

Anthelmintic resistance is a natural and inevitable consequence of drug treatment. As long as chemical control remains a feature of parasite management, we will be selecting for resistance in target parasite populations. Increasing levels of anthelmintic resistance in the coming years are virtually assured. The first reports of total treatment failure against cyathostomins or *Parascaris* spp. may be just a few years away. Once this knowledge is publicized, the horse-owning public will demand radical changes, and the veterinary profession must be equipped to respond.

No biological rationale can assume that large strongyles or tapeworms are also incapable of developing anthelmintic resistance. The most likely explanations for its delayed appearance include longer life cycles, which protract the generation interval, and the high efficacy of larvicidal treatments. Anthelmintic resistance in a highly pathogenic parasite like *Strongylus vulgaris* would constitute a very serious threat to equine health.

New anthelmintics?

At some point in the future, the pharmaceutical industry will introduce new anthelmintic drugs to the equine market. However, these pending products will differ from their predecessors in many important ways. First, they are not likely to be as efficacious as the macrocyclic lactones. Drugs with such exceptional efficacy, safety, and breadth of spectrum only come along once in a generation. Second, new anthelmintics will be far more expensive than currently available dewormers and manufacturers should give serious consideration to marketing these products on a strictly ethical basis, forgoing over-the-counter sales. These measures should be implemented to leverage greater veterinary involvement in parasite control programs and, if for no other reason, to dissuade casual abuse by horse owners (As of 2017, it is possible to purchase a dose of generic ivermectin paste to deworm a 500 kg adult horse for a retail cost of less than US$3). Third, these products must be used more wisely and in a sustainable fashion. If new compounds are abused as blatantly as their ancestors, eventual resistance is assured. With this in mind, we can only hope that commercial manufacturers will change their advertising strategies to promote sustainable use and thereby support the longevity of their product in the market place.

Of course, incorporating new anthelmintics into customized control strategies will depend on a number of factors, such as parasite spectrum (both species and stage of development), egg reappearance period, risk of adverse reactions, and cost of treatment. Regardless, the basic recommendations presented in this book are not likely to change just because a new drug has been introduced. Responsible use to maintain high efficacy will be paramount for any new or existing products.

It may also be tempting to combine two or more anthelmintics in a single treatment episode in an attempt to improve efficacy and to make use of drug formulations that would otherwise not be useful. As discussed in Chapter 7, this may be of value, but the success of this approach depends largely on the starting efficacies of each anthelmintic component and the utilization of horse *refugia* by leaving a proportion of the herd untreated.

Ten commandments

One take-home message from this book is that parasite control is not as simple as we would all like it to be, and that generic guidelines cannot be formulated for satisfactory control in all members of a herd. We recognize how frustrating this message must be for many people in the field, given the historical reliance on overly simplistic approaches. Just being told that things are complicated is not an effective agent of change. While it is almost impossible to give general advice on choice and timing of anthelmintic treatment on horse farms, it is very feasible to formulate a set of rules regarding "what not to do". We call this the Ten Commandments of Equine Parasite Control:

1) *Don't use an anthelmintic without knowing its efficacy against the intended parasite population.*
   The prevalence and intensity of anthelmintic resistance have become so great that none of the anthelmintic drugs

can be assumed to have 100% efficacy in every circumstance. The absolute starting point for all treatment regimens is to routinely evaluate the efficacy of available drugs.

2) *Don't treat at fixed intervals year-round.*
   Transmission of parasites is a biological system, and its intensity fluctuates with the seasons, the susceptibility of host populations, and innumerable other details. Although it may be easier to remember, it is totally illogical to implement parasite control as a regularly scheduled transaction, like a mortgage payment.

3) *Don't rotate blindly between anthelmintic drugs.*
   Anthelmintic drugs differ in their antiparasitic spectra, and one drug cannot be substituted blindly with a different product. The choice of drug depends on which parasite species are present and the goal of the treatment. Contrary to conventional wisdom, there is no scientific proof that drug rotation delays the development of resistance.

4) *Don't treat adult horses during the season when environmental translation is minimal (unless there is a clear clinical indication to do so).*
   If parasite transmission is controlled during the seasons of active translation, treatments outside this interval are unnecessary. In nearly every climate, there are substantial intervals during the year when environmental conditions are unfavorable for parasite transmission, and anthelmintic treatments at those times are potentially harmful. Strongyles are the major parasites of adult horses and they adhere to this rule very closely.

5) *Don't treat the entire herd just prior to a move to clean pasture.*
   The traditional "treat-and-move" strategy is now discouraged because it contradicts current knowledge about the

importance of parasite *refugia*. Clean pastures harbor minimal *refugia* and the first eggs to contaminate this new venue will all be produced by worms that survived the recent deworming. This practice introduces strong selection pressure for the development of anthelmintic resistance.

6) *Don't treat at the first frost.*

Although butterflies and dandelions disappear in winter, frost does not kill strongylid L_3s or ascarid eggs. As outlined in Commandment 4, winter treatments in a northern temperate climate are unnecessary, and could even introduce some risk of triggering larval cyathostominosis.

7) *Don't intentionally under-dose any anthelmintic treatment.*

Under-dosing has been identified as a definite risk factor for the development of anthelmintic resistance. Pharmaceutical companies and the regulatory agencies take considerable pains to ensure that the label dosage of any product is both safe and effective. Under-dosing carries no assurance of efficacy and its intentional implementation by a medical professional is irresponsible.

8) *Don't use anthelmintic formulations that are not labeled for horses or administer them by a route that is inconsistent with label directions.*

The pharmacokinetics and metabolism of drug formulations intended for administration to other animal species or via other routes of entry are generally unknown, so accurate dosages cannot be extrapolated. This practice introduces considerable risk of under-dosing and the possibility of illegal drug resides when employed for food animals.

9) *Don't ever just guess a horse's weight.*

While guessing a horse's weight is possible with reasonable accuracy after some training, it remains very difficult with foals, young horses, and ponies. It is our experience that even experienced horse owners and veterinarians can be off by over 100 kg in their estimates. Thus, it is important to verify body weights with either scales or a weight tape.

10) *Don't assume that all horses within a herd are heavily parasitized just because one animal developed parasitic disease.*

Parasite burdens are always unevenly distributed within a herd of horses, so a majority of herd members are likely to harbor small to moderate burdens. Furthermore, parasitic disease typically occurs in individuals that might be suffering from other concurrent issues.

Clinical cases for self-assessment

The 22 cases included in this book were carefully chosen to assess the reader's knowledge about equine parasites and to illustrate and demonstrate the concepts presented in the previous chapters. Each case history is accompanied by three or more questions, which are followed by suggested answers. We recognize that a typical reader may not read this book from beginning to end and may just select chapters or sections that are relevant to a current clinical challenge. A busy clinician might even prefer to start out with the cases, and we certainly welcome this approach. If you know all the answers, you will not need to read the book. If you don't, then each case will guide you to the relevant chapter for review. However, if you are reading this paragraph, you have probably already read the entire book. Regardless, enjoy.

Section IV

Case Histories

Case 1

Mystery Drug

History

A new client has a group of five Thoroughbred yearling colts that are being prepared for sale. Your partner dewormed this group about three weeks ago (~March 1) and based her anthelmintic selection on the results of pre-treatment fecal exams. You recall that she had to go back the day after deworming to treat one of the colts for a mild colic.

The post-treatment FECR results have landed in your mail box by mistake, so you accept the intellectual challenge of figuring out which dewormer she used (Table C1.1) You might also try to deduce a thing or two about the resistance status of the herd.

Table C1.1 Pre- and post-treatment fecal egg count results following treatment with an unknown equine anthelmintic.

Horse ID	Strongyles*		Parascaris*		Anoplocephala[†]	
	Pre-treatment	Post-treatment	Pre-treatment	Post-treatment	Pre-treatment	Post-treatment
A	825	250	175	25	63	0
B	900	350	125	0	47	0
C[‡]	500	250	325	25	22	0
D	1275	375	250	0	103	0
E	450	100	250	0	7	0

*McMaster; sensitivity 25 EPG.
[†]Modified Wisconsin technique, 1 EPG.
[‡]The lab record noted that 2 bots were found in the feces when submitted.

Questions

1 Which anthelmintic did she use? Can you deduce anything else about the anthelmintic susceptibility status of this herd?

2 What do you make of the bot stragglers?

Handbook of Equine Parasite Control, Second Edition. Martin K. Nielsen and Craig R. Reinemeyer.
© 2018 John Wiley & Sons, Inc. Published 2018 by John Wiley & Sons, Inc.

Answers

1 Let's go through the options in an organized fashion, and rule in or rule out the various classes.

Benzimidazoles. The treatment failed to achieve ≥90% efficacy against strongyles, so cyathostomin resistance must be a feasible characteristic of the mystery drug. Cyathostomin resistance to BZs is extremely common, plus the treatment was effective against adult ascarids. These features both support the historical use of a BZ such as fenbendazole or oxibendazole. However, the BZs have no efficacy against tapeworms, so we can assume that this drug class wasn't used.

Macrocyclic lactones. This class generally exhibits good efficacy against strongyles, but encounters high levels of resistance in ascarids. In addition, ivermectin or moxidectin have no cestocidal properties, so this class cannot explain the removal of tapeworms. But wait! There are....

Macrocyclic lactones combined with praziquantel. Praziquantel (PRZ) is an extremely effective cestocide, and several combinations of PRZ plus ivermectin or moxidectin are commercially available. The use of one of these products would explain the observed efficacy against tapeworms, but MLs rarely reduce ascarid egg counts very effectively anymore, and resistance to the extent exhibited in these strongyle egg counts has not been reported. Hopefully this is still many years away.

Pyrimidines. The pyrantel salts are broad spectrum dewormers, so they exhibit good efficacy against strongyles and ascarids. The mystery treatment did a good job against *Parascaris*, but the removal of strongyles was inadequate, and likely indicates resistance. This is quite feasible because pyrantel-resistant cyathostomins are widely reported across the world (Chapter 8). However, does pyrantel have any efficacy against tapeworms? Indeed, one pyrantel pamoate paste formulation is labeled for efficacy against *Anoplocephala perfoliata* when administered at 13.2 mg/kg. At the standard nematocidal dosage (6.6 mg/kg), pyrantel pamoate removed 80% or more of adult cestodes in controlled efficacy trials (see Chapter 7).

Therefore, you've not only identified the mystery drug, but you recognize that the herd in question probably harbors pyrantel-resistant cyathostomins. Also, ascarid impactions or obstructive colics are more common after treatment with anthelmintics that have a neuromuscular mode of action (see Chapter 7), so this item of historical trivia is also consistent with your product identification.

2 The bots were probably passing out of the host as a normal, seasonal phenomenon. Three weeks post-dosing is far too late to be a consequence of treatment. In addition, the fact that bots are still present three weeks after treatment is further evidence that macrocyclic lactones were not used.

Case 2

Pyrantel Efficacy Evaluation

History

A horse owner has sought your assistance to test for anthelmintic resistance against a pyrantel paste formulation on his Standardbred farm. He has used this drug regularly over the past ten years, and now wants to determine whether resistance has developed. You perform a fecal egg count reduction test (FECRT) and generate the data presented in Table C2.1.

Table C2.1 Strongylid fecal egg counts from a Standardbred herd, measured before and 14 days after treatment with pyrantel pamoate paste.

Pre-treatment	Post-treatment
300	0
300	20
780	0
520	0
340	0
400	60
260	0
280	40
860	140
400	80
300	0
200	120
300	20
640	40

Handbook of Equine Parasite Control, Second Edition. Martin K. Nielsen and Craig R. Reinemeyer.
© 2018 John Wiley & Sons, Inc. Published 2018 by John Wiley & Sons, Inc.

Questions

1 What is the calculated FECR for this farm?

   A What is your interpretation of the result?

2 What is your recommendation for this farm regarding the future use of pyrantel products?

Answers

1 The FECRT is calculated in Table C2.2, using guidelines presented in Chapter 10. A simple estimate of the

Table C2.2 Calculation of FECRT results for the farm.

Pre-treatment	Post-treatment
300	0
300	20
780	0
520	0
340	0
400	60
260	0
280	40
860	140
400	80
300	0
200	120
300	20
640	40
5880	520
FECR (%)	91.16

FECR is achieved by calculating total pre- and post-treatment FECs for this group and then calculating the percent reduction. Thus, the calculation in this case will be $(1 - (5880 - 520)/5880) \times 100\% = \textbf{91\%}$.

   A This result is inconclusive. Although the FECR is numerically above 90%, these results fall in the gray zone, wherein the influence of chance variability cannot be excluded. Therefore, it is recommended that the FECRT be repeated for this farm.

2 Horses would benefit from a 91% reduction of egg shedding, so the drug can be used on the farm. However, if the true efficacy is less than indicated by these samples, resistance may be accelerated if this drug is used frequently or exclusively. Recommendations would be to retest pyrantel's efficacy, as mentioned above, and possibly use a drug with a higher efficacy.

Case 3

Egg Count Results from Yearlings

History

A herd of pastured yearlings from northern Illinois was screened for possible enrollment in an anthelmintic field trial. Farm employees were not familiar with any details regarding recent anthelmintic treatment, but those records could be supplied by the stable manager when he returns from vacation. The following fecal diagnostic results were reported (Table C3.1).

Table C3.1 Quantitative fecal egg count results, Big Ridge Stables.

Horse I.D.	Parascaris*	Strongyles*	Anoplocephala*
A	456	0	17
B	1019	0	3
C	0	0	0
D	177	0	25
E	342	0	137
F	556	0	88
G	412	0	76
H	30	0	0
I	601	0	33
J	18	0	60

*All results reported as eggs per gram.

Questions

1 How can one determine that the quantitative fecal examination procedure used was NOT the McMaster's technique?

2 What are the two most unusual features of these fecal results?

3 Of these two unusual features, which is clearly a consequence of pasture-based management?

4 What is the only explanation for the other anomaly?

Handbook of Equine Parasite Control, Second Edition. Martin K. Nielsen and Craig R. Reinemeyer.
© 2018 John Wiley & Sons, Inc. Published 2018 by John Wiley & Sons, Inc.

5   The prevalence and magnitude of ascarid egg counts allow one to define the specific management intervention that was identified by question 4. What was it?

6   What future recommendations might you provide for helminth management in this herd?

Answers

1   The McMaster's is a dilution technique in which the raw egg counts (*numbers of eggs actually observed microscopically and counted*) are multiplied by a standard conversion factor to generate final egg counts (*expressed as eggs per gram*). For example, a McMaster technique using 4 grams of feces and 26 ml of flotation solution has a standard conversion factor of 25 (Chapter 9). Thus, all of the positive egg counts from a similar McMaster technique would be divisible by 25. The egg counts in this series have no common denominator >1.

2   A Unusually high prevalence of positive results for tapeworms (*Anoplocephala*).
    B Total absence of positive strongyle egg counts.

3   *Anoplocephala* infections are transmitted by ingestion of free-living oribatid mites, which occur almost exclusively in forage-based management systems. In contrast, ascarids can be acquired from stable or paddock habitats.

4   It is virtually unheard of for an entire pastured herd of young horses to have strongyle egg counts of "0". The only logical explanation is recent treatment with an anthelmintic that exhibits high efficacy against strongyles.

5   If anthelmintic therapy is the only explanation for consistent "0" strongyle egg counts, then treatment must have involved a drug that concurrently spares tapeworms and ascarids.

One can rule out any anthelmintic combination containing praziquantel, which has virtually 100% efficacy against cestodes (plus, the prepatent period for *Anoplocephala* is much longer than the reappearance period of strongyle eggs). One could probably also exclude any treatment involving pyrantel products because they also have some efficacy against cestodes. In addition, pyrantel would be unlikely to reduce strongylid egg counts to zero in all treated horses.

This leaves only benzimidazoles, piperazine, and macrocyclic lactones as alternative explanations. Piperazine exhibits good efficacy against ascarids, but only modest activity against strongyles. The benzimidazoles and macrocyclic lactones are both broad spectrum drugs, with efficacy against ascarids and strongyles. In this case, the operative drug clearly worked against only a single target population – strongyles. How can one explain the lack of efficacy against *Parascaris*?

The farm manager was contacted relative to these results, and he was able to confirm that all yearlings had been dewormed two weeks previously with ivermectin paste. Clearly, the ascarid population on this farm was resistant to macrocyclic lactone anthelmintics, although the indigenous strongyles were obviously susceptible. See Chapters 7 and 8 for an overview of the different anthelmintics and their efficacy levels.

6 See Chapter 12 for a discussion of ascarid management in herds with known macrocyclic lactone resistance. The high prevalence of *Anoplocephala* eggs indicates that regular cestode control measures are warranted. Biannual treatments (spring and autumn) with praziquantel or pyrantel pamoate (13.2 mg/kg) should be recommended.

(Note: In the authors' experience, a high prevalence of patent *Anoplocephala* infections in a herd may indicate the presence of *A. magna* or mixed infections, rather than *A. perfoliata* alone. Management recommendations would be identical.)

Case 4

Peritonitis and Parasites

History

An 8 year old Icelandic stallion used for breeding and competition riding collapsed at an event with signs of colic. A veterinarian present at the event examined the horse and found it in lateral recumbency with cyanotic mucous membranes and a heart rate of 80 beats per minute. She referred the stallion to a university hospital for further management. Following admission, the horse responded well to pain management, but continued to have decreased intestinal peristalsis and exhibited very limited appetite. An abdominocentesis revealed clear signs of peritonitis and an exploratory laparotomy was performed. Surgeons found a circular devitalized area of the ventral colon. The area was accompanied by a stricture of the intestine, with fibrous adhesions to the abdominal wall. The devitalized and strictured intestine was resected and adhesions were broken down. Recovery was slow but uneventful.

The owner was informed that the lesion could have originated as parasitic damage. She admitted that her horses had not been dewormed at all during the past year. She owns a small stud farm and is now worried that her horses might suffer from serious parasite infection. None are showing any signs of parasitism, but she asks her local veterinarian to collect fecal samples from all horses on the premises and perform fecal egg counts and larval cultures. The results are presented in Table C4.1. Figure C4.1 depicts some of the non-cyathostomin larvae that were observed.

Handbook of Equine Parasite Control, Second Edition. Martin K. Nielsen and Craig R. Reinemeyer.
© 2018 John Wiley & Sons, Inc. Published 2018 by John Wiley & Sons, Inc.

Table C4.1 Results of fecal egg counts and larval cultures for all horses on a farm. Larval culture results are presented as the total number of non-cyathostomin larvae encountered in the sample.

Age of horse	Fecal egg count	Non-cyathostomin larvae
16	40	0
18	0	4
10	20	0
5	240	6
10	380	5
4	1000	26
21	120	0
1	160	0
1	2300	121
2	960	37
4	200	2
2	440	6
31	1340	3
14	640	54
8	180	0
1	1600	27
10	60	0
10	120	1
7	0	0

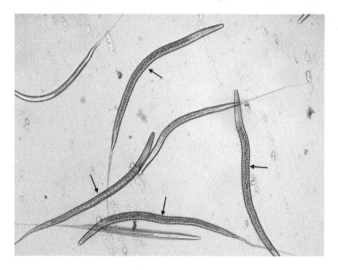

Figure C4.1 Non-cyathostomin larvae encountered in larval cultures (arrows).

Questions

1 Which strongyle species do you recognize in Figure C4.1?

2 Which anthelmintic drugs would you expect to be efficacious against these parasites?

3 What anthelmintic treatment strategy do you recommend on the farm?

Answers

1 The smaller larvae in the picture are cyathostomins and are characterized by filamentous tails and eight intestinal cells. The larvae indicated by arrows are *Strongylus vulgaris*. They are larger than the cyathostomin larvae present, and definitive identification is provided by the presence of 28 to 32 intestinal cells.

2 All broad spectrum equine anthelmintics have good efficacy against adult *S. vulgaris*. However, they are not all effective against migrating stages. The macrocyclic lactones are effective against younger migrating stages. Fenbendazole can kill migrating larvae as well, but only if administered at an elevated dosage for five consecutive days. Pyrantel only has activity against luminal intestinal stages.

3 Several options are available for this farm, depending on their goals. In this case, the most important goal is to reduce the presence of *Strongylus vulgaris* to a negligible level. The owner must recognize that eradication is not feasible, but that large strongyles can be reduced to a level where they are encountered in low numbers in just a few horses. Another relevant goal would be to reduce egg shedding for the entire farm.

It would be relevant to discuss management procedures with the owner, especially the quality and availability of pastures. If the owner is motivated, pasture hygiene can be recommended to reduce the infection pressure.

For anthelmintic treatments, the basic foundation should include larvicidal applications that are sufficiently frequent to disrupt the life cycle of *S. vulgaris*. As the prepatent period is about six months, two treatments applied to all horses and spaced at equal intervals during the annual cycle should reduce the occurrence considerably. Egg counts should be evaluated at least once annually to identify the high, moderate, and low egg shedders. Larval cultures can be performed in the spring at the onset of the grazing season to detect large strongyle infections.

A few additional treatments should be considered for foals that are at risk of acquiring *Parascaris* spp. burdens. See Chapter 12 for a discussion of parasite control strategies.

Case 5

Confinement after Deworming

History

You are contacted by the owner of a riding school with 80 adult horses and ponies. For many years, they have practiced meticulous, regular deworming of the entire herd. As a routine post-deworming procedure, all horses are held in their stalls for five days before being turned out to pastures. During this confinement period, personnel remove all manure and replace the bedding. This measure is labor-intensive and expensive, so she wants to know whether shortening the period to three days would present any risks.

Questions

1   Identify the risks of parasite transmission, if any, during the post-treatment period. Which parasites are in question, and why are they a risk during the post-treatment period?

2   Describe potential adverse reactions to anthelmintic treatment that any horse might experience. What is the likely post-treatment interval during which most of these adverse events would occur?

3   Considering your answers to questions 1 and 2, how would you respond to the owner's query about an abbreviated interval?

Answers

1   The rationale behind this confinement procedure is unclear, and isn't really very logical. The primary parasites in adult horses are strongyles, and possibly tapeworms and pinworms. *Parascaris* spp. is unlikely to occur in mature horses. It is important to remind the client that the strongyle eggs that are passed in the feces are not infective until they have hatched and developed into infective third stage larvae (Chapter 3). Horses with positive egg counts shed thousands of parasite eggs every day, and this contamination gradually declines to a very low level during the days following an efficacious treatment. Thus, the amount of eggs contributed during the few days post-treatment will be negligible compared to the parasite egg output on pasture during the weeks or months prior to the treatment.

Handbook of Equine Parasite Control, Second Edition. Martin K. Nielsen and Craig R. Reinemeyer.
© 2018 John Wiley & Sons, Inc. Published 2018 by John Wiley & Sons, Inc.

Dead worms are always expelled after deworming, but only the larger of these are visible to the naked eye. Regardless, adult worms are not infective to the horses, even if some of them were still alive.

Tapeworm eggs have been found to be more abundant in the feces following treatment with a tapeworm drug in horses (see Chapter 9). However, it is important to remember that the life cycle involves development within oribatid mites before horses can become infected. It is unknown whether these mites occur in stalls, but the risk of tapeworm infection in stables must be considered to be minor. The only other possible justification for this practice is the theoretical risk of eggs contained within the uteri of treated female worms being able to develop into the infective stage. For strongyle parasites this must be considered unlikely because a majority of these eggs would be immature and not yet fully developed. In addition, the worm would have to disintegrate for the eggs to make it to the environment, and daily removal would obviate that risk as well.

The best theoretical justification for the confinement procedure would be for *Parascaris* spp. in foals. A female ascarid contains hundreds of thousands of eggs. Given their ability to resist environment influences, a share of these eggs are likely to remain viable even after the death of the worm. However, the riding school in question only has adult horses.

2   Post-dosing reactions involve non-specific colics, transient diarrheas, and larval cyathostominosis (see Chapter 7). Although these are more likely to occur in younger horses, chances are that some of the 80 horses at this riding school may encounter such reactions. It is therefore advisable to monitor horses for these reactions. However, this does not necessarily involve stall confinement. The choice of observation period is also unclear. Most of the milder reactions occur within the first few days, but one study showed that anthelmintic treatment constituted a risk factor for larval cyathostominosis during the following two weeks.

3   As outlined above, this confinement procedure makes very little sense, and we see no reason to continue it. Disinfection measures are not justified, and are generally ineffective anyhow. At most, the owner and her personnel should be instructed about the small risk of adverse reactions to anthelmintic treatment.

Case 6

Abdominal Distress in a Foal

History

A 5 month old Trakhener filly was orphaned at birth and hand-raised in confinement. The foal had received tetanus antitoxin after birth, but no additional vaccines or anthelmintic treatments in the interim.

In late August, the foal developed colic of 5 hours' duration. The referring veterinarian classified the pain as severe, and treatment with opioid analgesics provided only transient relief. The foal was referred to a tertiary care center.

Clinical assessment

The foal presented with abdominal distention; mucous membranes were hyperemic with a CRT of three seconds; heart rate 40 BPM; respiratory rate 20 BPM. Manifestations of colic were manageable with xylazine and metamizole, and gastric reflux was absent. Abdominal ultrasound revealed a distended small intestine with hyperechogenic, linear, motile objects within the lumen (Figure C6.1).

Laboratory findings

Hemogram: normal
Serum chemistry: unremarkable
Abdominocentesis: 10 g protein/L and
                   $<10^9$ leukocytes/L
McMaster   480 strongyle EPG;
Quantitative Egg   80 *Parascaris* EPG
Count:

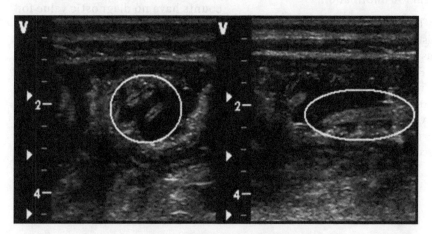

Figure C6.1 Transabdominal ultrasound of the small intestine of a foal with colic. Several hyperechogenic, linear objects were identified in the lumen (circled). The figure depicts transverse (left) and longitudinal (right) sections of the intraluminal objects.

Handbook of Equine Parasite Control, Second Edition. Martin K. Nielsen and Craig R. Reinemeyer.
© 2018 John Wiley & Sons, Inc. Published 2018 by John Wiley & Sons, Inc.

Questions

1 What is the most likely clinical diagnosis?
  A Other differential diagnoses?

2 What specific, antiparasitic treatment plan would you recommend for this foal?

3 The owners operate a small Trakhener breeding operation. What general recommendations would you make to prevent similar recurrences in future foals?

Answers

1 Small intestinal impaction with *Parascaris* spp. Other causes of small intestinal obstruction, such as volvulus or epiploic entrapment.

2 The foal was treated with one dose of fenbendazole paste (7.5 mg/kg) to minimize the risk of exacerbating the impaction (see Chapter 7 for a discussion of anthelmintics with a paralytic mode of action); 7.5 mg/kg is the label dosage for *Parascaris* spp. in Europe, while it is 10 mg/kg in North America. The slower onset of effect of this drug class should decrease the risk of exacerbating the impaction. There is likely no value in reducing the dose as even half the dose should be just as effective.

Additional clinical information

In addition to fenbendazole, mineral oil was administered via a nasogastric tube. The foal was monitored closely for the 24 hours after FBZ treatment and evaluated for gastric reflux at 3 hour intervals. Approximately 40 dead ascarids were recovered via gastric intubation, and worms were observed passing in the feces from the second day following treatment.

The foal was sent home five days after admission.

3 It is advisable to deworm foals at about 2–3 months of age to prevent accumulation of large burdens of *Parascaris* spp. (see Chapter 12). In consideration of the current levels of resistance to ivermectin/moxidectin and the risk of impaction associated with paralytic anthelmintics, benzimidazoles may be the best choice for this treatment. A second ascarid-directed treatment is generally recommended around 5 months of age, and preferably before weaning. In most cases, this should be followed up by a strongyle- and possibly tapeworm-directed treatment at around 6 months of age. Fecal egg counts have no diagnostic value for foals that are younger than the pre-patent period of *Parascaris* (*i.e.*, approximately 3 months), but can be useful for evaluating treatment efficacy and for monitoring the relative levels of ascarids and strongyles in older juveniles (see Chapter 9 for a discussion of diagnostic methods).

Case 7

Quarantining Advice

History

A client just bought a new, adult mare and asks for your advice. She owns a small, Arabian breeding operation and doesn't want to introduce "bad parasites" into her herd. She reports that clinical parasitism has never been a problem on her property and she intends to keep it that way. Her

initial plan is to quarantine the new horse on an isolated paddock before introducing it into the herd, but she has a couple of questions for you:

1) Which dewormer should she use for the new horse?
2) How long should she quarantine the horse?

Questions

1 Before attempting to answer her questions, she needs to define the potential goals of the intended quarantine. Which "bad" parasites should she be intent on avoiding?

2 For each of these, how would you prevent their introduction on to the farm?

3 Based on these requirements, do you concur with her desire to quarantine the horse?

Answers

1 The point of any quarantine measure is to prevent the introduction of parasites (or genetically selected populations thereof) that are currently absent from the farm. Even without performing any fecal examinations, one can safely assume that her herd already harbors cyathostomins. *Parascaris* spp. are likely to be present in the foals and yearlings in residence and *Anoplocephala perfoliata* would not be unexpected for a pasture-based management system. In general, two

parasite categories are considered undesirable on any farm: (a) large strongyles, especially *Strongylus vulgaris*, because of its pathogenic potential, and (b) drug-resistant populations of cyathostomins and/or *Parascaris*.

2 The large strongyles are relatively simple to manage, because anthelmintic resistance is not an issue with this group. For effective management, one should choose drugs with efficacy against both luminal and migrating

Handbook of Equine Parasite Control, Second Edition. Martin K. Nielsen and Craig R. Reinemeyer.
© 2018 John Wiley & Sons, Inc. Published 2018 by John Wiley & Sons, Inc.

stages, which rules out piperazine, pyrantel, and single-dose benzimidazoles. Avoiding anthelmintic resistance is much more difficult. Fecal egg count reduction testing (FECRT) permits evaluation of only one drug at a time and is best performed when a horse is shedding moderate to high numbers of eggs. Especially relevant to the current case, FECRT is of limited value when performed on only one horse, and the results should be interpreted with great caution. The most pragmatic approach for quarantine is to test the efficacy of whichever drug is used most commonly on the farm. In most cases, this will likely be ivermectin.

3 Quarantining has the most value if one possesses solid information about the current parasite status of the farm. For instance, if large strongyles were already present, eliminating them from a new arrival has little value. Similarly, knowing the efficacy status of various anthelmintic classes against indigenous parasites helps to determine the best diagnostic information that can be gleaned from the new horse.

Case 8

Diarrhea and Colic

History

A 7 month old, grade colt, 215 kg, was dewormed with an unknown product two months ago. Since that time, the foal has lost weight, and developed a rough haircoat and "tucked up" appearance. Feces were soft to watery and preputial edema was observed. When admitted on January 1, the foal had experienced recurrent, mild colic for the past four weeks. The referring vet had been called to examine the colt on several occasions and had treated it with opioids for pain, sulfa+trimethoprim antibiotics, and non-steroidal anti-inflammatory drugs.

Clinical assessment

The foal had clear manifestations of pain, with constant rolling. The heart rate was within the normal range, and mucous membranes were pink with a capillary refill time of 3 seconds. Slight ventral edema was noted in the sternal area. Transabdominal ultrasound revealed an abnormal appearance of the cecum with unusual, hyperechogenic areas. Feces ranged from loose to normal in consistency.

Laboratory findings

WBCC:	20.07×10^9 cells/l (leukocytosis)
Neutrophils:	17.32×10^9 cells/l (absolute neutrophilia) (86.3%)
Total protein:	38.98 g/l (hypoproteinemia)
Albumin:	22.38 g/l (hypoalbuminemia)
Abdominal tap:	0.55×10^9 cells/l with protein 2 g/l (normal)
Blood and feces for *Lawsonia intracellularis*:	negative
Bacterial cultures for *Salmonella* and *Clostridium* spp.:	negative
McMaster Quantitative Fecal Egg Count:	40 strongyle EPG
Direct Baermann for cyathostomin larvae:	negative

Treatment

The clinicians had no primary suspicion of a parasitic problem and were focused on managing the colic. Pain could not be

Handbook of Equine Parasite Control, Second Edition. Martin K. Nielsen and Craig R. Reinemeyer.
© 2018 John Wiley & Sons, Inc. Published 2018 by John Wiley & Sons, Inc.

controlled with the panel of analgesics available, so a laparotomy was performed on January 5. The cecum had an invagination involving ~ 50% of the organ wall. The affected portion of the cecum was resected and unaffected portions of the large intestinal wall were found to be extremely edematous. Regional lymph nodes were markedly enlarged. After surgery, the colt was treated with intravenous fluids, lidocaine infusion, meloxicam, metronidazole, cefquinome, and omeprazole.

Questions

1 Which parasitic condition is the most likely cause of the case described herein? Which factors support this diagnosis?

   A What diagnostic measures can be applied to reach a definitive diagnosis?

2 Which anthelmintics should be considered for managing this condition?

3 What other equine parasite could cause the surgical condition described above?

Answers

1 Larval cyathostominosis should be suspected because of the following factors: the time of year, immature age of the host, historical loss of weight and body condition, loose feces, ventral edema, hypoproteinemia, leukocytosis, and a history of deworming prior to the onset of clinical signs. It is somewhat unusual to encounter this condition at this age, as foals generally do not graze extensively during their first summer and acquire relatively small burdens of encysted worms. However, larval cyathostominosis has been reported in weanlings. The bacterial infection *Lawsonia intracellularis* is an important differential diagnosis in this age group and can cause similar signs. Some case studies have reported intussusceptions and cecal invaginations associated with larval cyathostominosis.

   A No reliable diagnostic tests are available for diagnosing larval cyathostominosis. The direct Baermann method employed here represents an attempt to identify recently emerged cyathostomin larvae in the feces, but this procedure probably has low diagnostic sensitivity. This is discussed further in Chapter 9.

   B In the present case, histopathology of a sample of resected tissue might have revealed severe inflammation associated with high numbers of encysted larvae.

2 Moxidectin should be considered for treating a clinical case of larval cyathostominosis (see Chapter 7). This drug appears to cause minimal inflammatory reaction and its efficacy against encysted cyathostomins is not compromised by potential resistance issues.

3 Tapeworms (*Anoplocephala perfoliata*) can cause spastic and mechanical colics related to the cecal region. The latter can be attributed to ileal impactions, cecocolic intussusceptions, and, possibly, cecal invagination. Tapeworm infection causes inflammation and edema of the cecal wall, but lesions are generally restricted to

the immediate vicinity of attachment sites. However, hypoproteinemia and hypoalbuminemia, as observed in this case, have not been associated with tapeworm infection.

A A modified egg counting technique can be applied for *Anoplocephala* diagnosis. ELISA techniques for detecting antibodies are also options, but a positive result may indicate historical exposure rather than contemporaneous infection (see Ch. 9).

Outcome

After initially improving for approximately two weeks post-surgery, colic signs resumed and the horse was euthanatized on February 1. At necropsy, regional parasitic typhlocolitis (*i.e.*, larval cyathostominosis) was diagnosed, and myriad, vacated, parasitic cysts were visualized in the mucosal lining, along with marked edema of the large intestinal walls and enlarged regional lymph nodes.

Case 9

Foal Diarrhea

History

A Morgan horse breeding facility foaled approximately one dozen mares this spring. The mares foal in individual stalls, and mares and foals are turned out to a communal pasture about 7 days post-partum. The foal crop is doing well although virtually 100% of them experienced foal heat diarrhea (FHD) beginning during the second week of life. All foals recovered uneventfully within the next week or two. One colt (Ajax, born to a primiparous mare that had been purchased the previous year) developed watery diarrhea beginning at 31 days of age.

Clinical assessment

The foal now suckles less frequently than expected and seems slightly lethargic. Ajax's physical exam reveals slight dehydration, and the perineum and hindquarters have been "scalded" by diarrhea. Watery, khaki-colored feces were passed in response to introduction of a rectal thermometer, and a sample was collected for diagnostic testing. The rectal temperature was 39.1 °C (102.4 °F).

Diagnostics

Feces were submitted for a fecal flotation exam and bacterial culture. Bacterial cultures revealed none of the typical foal pathogens (*Salmonella, Clostridium*), but the fecal exam (performed the same day) revealed high numbers of the object depicted in Figure C9.1.

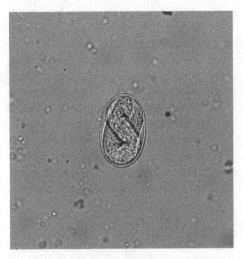

Figure C9.1 Parasite egg encountered in fecal samples.

Handbook of Equine Parasite Control, Second Edition. Martin K. Nielsen and Craig R. Reinemeyer.
© 2018 John Wiley & Sons, Inc. Published 2018 by John Wiley & Sons, Inc.

Questions

1 The lab results were: "larvated stron-gyle eggs". Provide at least two reasons why one should discount this diagnosis as erroneous.

2 What is the correct diagnosis?

3 What treatment would you prescribe? Prognosis?

4 Should fecal samples from other, healthy foals be examined? Is rote treatment of the foal herd warranted without individual diagnostics?

5 What are management recommen-dations for the mature members of the herd? For the stable facilities? For the pasture?

Answers

1 A The minimum prepatent period for any equine strongylid infection is 5.5 to 6 weeks. This foal is too young to harbor a mature infection.

   B Strongyle eggs larvate only in the presence of aerobic conditions and a temperature greater than 7.5 °C (45 °F). This sample was collected fresh and processed promptly, so even if strongyle eggs had been present, they would not have had adequate time to larvate.

   C It remains possible, however, that larvated strongyle eggs had been ingested via coprophagy and were recovered as false-positives. Hoever, if the eggs were measured or exam-ined closely, one might observe that they were smaller than the typical range for strongylid ova, were more round than elliptical, and had a thin shell.

2 *Strongyloides westeri* infection.

3 Treatment with either ivermectin (0.2 mg/kg) or oxibendazole (15 mg/kg). (Moxidectin is presumably effective, but is not labeled in the United States for use in foals less than 6 months of age.) The prognosis is excellent and

clinical signs normally disappear within 48 hours.

4 The need for additional fecal testing is equivocal. If additional positive foals were identified, specific ther-apy is nevertheless unnecessary as long as they remain clinically nor-mal. For the same reason, rote treat-ment is not advised, and any unnecessary use of anthelmintics can select for resistance in non-target nematode populations (in this case, *Parascaris*).

5 *Strongyloides* is an unusual nematode in that infection is ultimately con-trolled 100% by acquired immunity. Immunity is often fully effective by about 12 months of age, so mature ani-mals are not threatened at all by this parasitism. It was a common manage-ment practice to deworm mares dur-ing the last month of gestation with a macrocyclic lactone anthelmintic to prevent lactogenic transmission of *Strongyloides* from the mare to her suckling foal. The justification for this measure is questionable, given the low incidence of *Strongyloides* disease in foals.

Sanitation of foaling facilities for the prevention of *Strongyloides* is not necessary, as long as mares and foals don't reside therein for longer than one week. Infections can be transmitted by soiled bedding, particularly moist saw dust. This situation could arise if a two-week or older foal (with a patent *S. westeri* infection) had contaminated a stall or pen, and other foals subsequently occupied the same area.

It is virtually impossible to eradicate *S. westeri* from pasture habitats. *Strongyloides* can pass several generations in the environment as free-living populations, even in the total absence of horses on the premise. Attempts at eradication would be fruitless.

Case 10

Oral Lesion

History

A horse that had been salivating for several days is sedated and subjected to a thorough oral examination. The exam includes examination of oral structures with a flexible endoscope, with which you captured the image depicted in Figure C10.1.

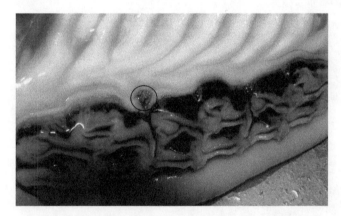

Figure C10.1 A larva (circled) is visible on the lingual border of a maxillary, interdental junction.

Questions

1 Which parasite is this most likely to be?

2 What is the pathogenic impact of this parasite?

3 Which treatment recommendations would you give to the owner?

Answers

1 The localization and appearance is consistent with bot larvae, likely of *Gasterophilus intestinalis*. As described in Chapter 1, first- and second-instar larvae reside in the oral cavity before they proceed to the stomach. Considering the extremely high prevalence of bots, this would not be an unusual

Handbook of Equine Parasite Control, Second Edition. Martin K. Nielsen and Craig R. Reinemeyer.
© 2018 John Wiley & Sons, Inc. Published 2018 by John Wiley & Sons, Inc.

finding in oral examinations conducted during the warmer months of the year.

2 Little is known about the pathogenic impact of bot larvae in the oral cavity, but they have been reported to cause excessive salivation, lingual irritation, and chewing problems (Chapter 2). It is now accepted that the life cycle stages attached to the gastric mucosa only rarely cause clinical disease.

3 Ivermectin has demonstrated efficacy against oral stages of bot larvae. Moxidectin is also likely to also possess some effect against oral stages, but the efficacy against gastric stages is known to be variable (Chapter 7), which makes this an uncertain choice. Horses probably profit very little from bot treatments. One potential benefit may be fewer adult flies to lay eggs in the successive grazing season. However, even then, one's bot control program is only as good as that of the neighbor.

Case 11

Skin Lesion

History

A 4 year old Arabian stallion from northern Indiana, USA, was treated twice last summer for a small laceration on the medial, left front pastern. The laceration was not discovered until it was a few days old, and no attempt was made to suture it. Within a few weeks, the site had developed exuberant granulation tissue. The "proud flesh" was trimmed and the lesion treated by standard methods once in mid-August and again in late September. The second treatment seemed more successful than the first, and the lesion shrank to minimal size (~4 mm × 14 mm) during winter. In early June the following year, the owner called to report that the lesion had returned and was larger than previously.

Clinical assessment

The skin lesion is ~3 cm × 5 cm and extends ~5 to 7 mm above the surface of the surrounding skin. The lesion is ulcerated and has a serosanguinous exudate. It is attracting flies and the stallion spends several minutes during each hour rubbing the lesion with its muzzle.

No other horses in the herd are affected. This stallion has received pyrantel tartrate on a daily basis for the past 2.5 years.

Diagnostics

McMaster Egg Count:	75 strongylid EPG
CBC:	WBCC 13.87 × 10^9 cells/l (slight leukocytosis)
Eosinophils:	2.93 × 10^9 cells/l (absolute eosinophilia)

Questions

1 What is the most likely parasitologic diagnosis?

2 How could you arrive at a definitive diagnosis?

3 What therapeutic plan would you pursue?

4 Should you examine fecal samples from other horses on the farm to determine whether they might be carriers of the offending organism?

Handbook of Equine Parasite Control, Second Edition. Martin K. Nielsen and Craig R. Reinemeyer.
© 2018 John Wiley & Sons, Inc. Published 2018 by John Wiley & Sons, Inc.

Answers

1 Cutaneous habronemiasis. Horses harbor three species of spirurid worms that reside as adults in the stomach. *Habronema muscae* is by far the most common. *H. microstoma* has never been very prevalent, and *Draschia megastoma* has become increasingly rare since the advent of macrocyclic lactone anthelmintics (Chapter 1). These nematodes require dipteran intermediate hosts, which apparently deposit the larvae on to fresh wounds or mucocutaneous junctions, where they can invade the dermis and cause local pathology as described here (Chapter 2).

2 The appearance of the lesion and accompanying exudates, pruritus, absolute eosinophilia, and regression of lesions during winter months are all typical for cutaneous habronemiasis (Chapter 2). Regardless, a definitive diagnosis requires biopsy of the lesion and histopathologic demonstration of nematode larvae in the tissues.

3 The larvicidal properties of systemic macrocyclic lactone treatment are often sufficient to effect a clinical cure. Systemic corticosteroids have been used with success, and daily bandaging with some combination of antibiotics, corticosteroids, organophosphates, or DMSO are helpful. Large lesions might require surgical debulking in addition to medical therapy.

4 Additional fecal testing would be fruitless. The egg stages of *Habronema* and *Draschia* are quite small and might not survive the flotation process. To eliminate other horses (albeit temporarily) as sources of spirurid larvae, the simplest approach would be to deworm them with ivermectin, which should be effective against gastric stages.

Alternate fate

You later discuss this case with a colleague, who mentions that she has been treating a similar horse for several months with little, if any, success.

Questions (2)

5 Is anthelmintic resistance a possibility?

6 Alternative recommendations for the problem case?

Answers (2)

5 Many practitioners report that some cutaneous habronemiasis lesions do not respond to anthelmintic therapy as predictably as they did 10 years ago (Chapter 8).

Although resistance to macrocyclic lactones has not been documented in spirurid nematodes of horses, it is biologically quite feasible. Gastric *Habronema* infections are fairly common, so this genus could be exposed to selection pressure when members of a herd are treated with ivermectin or moxidectin. Unfortunately, no antemortem tests are capable of demonstrating resistance in these worms. One would have to conduct a classic efficacy study involving a control group and post-mortem worm counts, and this has not been done thus far.

6 A lack of response to macrocyclic lactones might require one to dust off the pharmacopeia of antiquity. In the good old days, topical or systemic organophosphates were used, with varying success, against these dermal infections.

Case 12

Legal Case

History

A 1 year old pony was sold on the first of October in Denmark. The new owner decides to keep the pony in the stable of origin for another six months before she transfers it to her own facility on the first of April. On April 4 the new arrival develops profuse, watery diarrhea and clear manifestations of colic, with cyanotic mucous membranes and a heart rate of 80 to 100 beats per minute. Despite intensive fluid therapy and colic management, the pony does not recover and is euthanized. The attending veterinarian performed an autopsy and found that the cecal and ventral colonic mucosa were extremely edematous, and had numerous, pinpoint hemorrhagic lesions consistent with newly emerged cyathostomin larvae. The mucosal surfaces were hemorrhagic and inflamed, with areas of necrosis. Huge numbers of cyathostomin larvae and worms were found in the luminal contents. The veterinarian diagnosed this case as acute larval cyathostominosis. After consulting with her veterinarian, the owner decided to file a civil lawsuit against the seller of the horse, claiming that the pony had acquired the parasites before October 1 of the prior year.

The court calls you as an expert witness on equine parasite infections and proposes a number of specific questions. You are presented with the historical information shared previously; there is no mention of anthelmintic treatments.

Questions

1 Is it likely that the pony was already infected with strongyle parasites on October 1?
   A If yes, please explain how.
   B If no, please explain how the parasites could have been acquired between October 1 and April 1.

2 Would it have been possible to detect the parasite burden in question during a pre-purchase examination in September? Could any diagnostic method have detected this condition prior to the onset of disease on April 4?

3 Could the disease occurring on April 4 have been prevented or mitigated if the pony had been treated with an anthelmintic after October 1?

4 What role could transfer to a different facility and change of housing and feed have played as a predisposing factor for larval cyathostominosis?

Handbook of Equine Parasite Control, Second Edition. Martin K. Nielsen and Craig R. Reinemeyer.
© 2018 John Wiley & Sons, Inc. Published 2018 by John Wiley & Sons, Inc.

Answers

1   Yes, it is highly likely that the pony had acquired these strongyle parasites prior to October 1.

    A Strongyle parasites are ubiquitous, and the grazing season defines the time of transmission. In Denmark, the grazing season typically extends from May through October.

    B If the pony had access to pasture after October 1, some additional larvae could have been acquired. However, this remains unknown because no additional information regarding the length of the grazing season or contemporaneous anthelmintic treatments was supplied in the testimony.

2   Fecal egg counts do not reflect encysted parasite burdens and would have had no diagnostic value in the present case. Low plasma protein values could, in theory, support suspicion of a large, encysted cyathostomin burden, but no definitive tools exist for diagnosis of encysted cyathostomins.

3   No information was available regarding prior anthelmintic treatment of this pony. In general, anthelmintic treatments between October and March (*i.e.,* while large numbers of larvae are encysted) would have comprised a risk factor for larval cyathostominosis. However, an effective larvicidal treatment administered in the specified time period should have reduced the encysted burden considerably and, thus, reduced the risk of larval cyathostominosis.

4   The scientific literature has not identified stabling type and change of feed as risk factors for larval cyathostominosis. However, relocation is recognized as a potential stressor, as detailed in Chapter 4, and could theoretically pose a risk factor for the development of larval cyathostominosis.

Case 13

Repeated Egg Counts

History

The owner of a riding school contacts you in the spring for your advice regarding their parasite control program. The horses on this farm are all adults, ranging between 6 to 24 years of age, and several breeds are represented. Until recently, this farm had dewormed all horses at regular intervals year-round, but the owners had done some on-line research and were interested in changing to a program based on fecal egg count results. They expressed some skepticism about egg counts, because they had also read that repeated counts from the same horse "could jump all over the place". As a mutual learning exercise, you offer to perform three repeated egg counts from each horse to illustrate the variability to the owner. The results are presented in Table C13.1.

Table C13.1 Results of three repeated strongyle egg counts from individual horses.

Horse	FEC1	FEC2	FEC3	Horse	FEC1	FEC2	FEC3
A	60	20	20	P	40	60	40
B	0	0	0	Q	0	0	0
C	200	260	260	R	0	0	0
D	540	420	400	S	40	60	40
E	0	20	20	T	0	0	0
F	0	0	0	U	0	0	0
G	760	1060	680	V	0	20	20
H	0	0	0	W	0	40	20
I	0	0	60	X	60	20	0
J	80	0	60	Y	640	520	500
K	0	20	0	Z	1020	820	760
L	100	160	20	AA	0	0	0
M	100	80	40	BB	40	20	40
N	0	0	0	CC	20	0	20
O	0	0	0	DD	420	380	260
				EE	620	500	600

Handbook of Equine Parasite Control, Second Edition. Martin K. Nielsen and Craig R. Reinemeyer.
© 2018 John Wiley & Sons, Inc. Published 2018 by John Wiley & Sons, Inc.

Questions

1 The riding instructor is now even more skeptical about the reliability of fecal egg counts, and argues that it appears to be totally coincidental whether or not a certain horse should be treated. Interpret these results and explain your findings to the owner.

2 Based on these samples, recommend a complete, annual parasite control regimen for this farm.

Answers

1 The variability in egg counts is within the expected range (±50%) and no horses exhibited extreme variability. The overall distribution of egg counts is typical for adult horses, with the majority shedding ≤200 EPG. Only four of these horses (G, Y, Z, EE) would be classified as High Contaminators.

Although it may be a challenge to convince the riding instructor, a number of arguments should be made: (1) egg counts should always be interpreted within broad ranges, and adult horses are likely to return to these levels after treatment; (2) the results have the expected variability, and there is good consistency between repeated counts; (3) if 200 EPG were chosen as the cut-off value for treatment, categorical recommendations (*i.e.*, treatment versus no treatment) would not have changed for any of these horses between sequential egg counts; (4) although repeated egg counts can fluctuate just above or below the cut-off value, an adult horse is likely to tolerate a low to moderate worm burden without treatment. If the riding instructor is still skeptical, it is always possible to adjust the cut-off value.

2 The egg counts of this herd are not alarming. However, it should be remembered that riding schools often experience substantial turnover, so parasite levels can change quickly. As a basic foundation, this herd could receive one yearly treatment with a combination of praziquantel plus ivermectin or moxidectin to manage tapeworms and help prevent large strongyles. This treatment should be administered in the autumn. Additional treatments could be administered in the spring, based on fecal egg count results. A cut-off value in the range of 100 to 300 EPG should be identified, and horses exceeding this value should be treated with ivermectin. The six horses with the highest egg counts should be chosen to perform a yearly fecal egg count reduction test to monitor for ivermectin resistance. For these adult horses, additional anthelmintic treatments (*i.e.*, other than autumn and spring) are not likely to be necessary.

Case 14

Repeated Colic

History

Danish Warmblood, gelding, 11 years old, 471 kg.

This horse had recurrent episodes of mild colic and was hospitalized in September. The formal diagnosis was sand impaction of the cecum, which was confirmed by imaging. A contemporary, quantitative fecal result was 0 strongylid EPG, and blood work was unremarkable. The horse was treated symptomatically with analgesics and I/V fluids, and sent home after a few days with a daily *Psyllium* substitution to alleviate the sand impaction. In late January, the horse had two episodes of mild colic and was treated by a local practitioner. After a third episode of colic within five days, the horse was hospitalized for further evaluation and treatment. At the time of admission, the horse had not received anthelmintic treatment for the past eight months.

Presentation

The horse was depressed, with mildly to moderately painful colic. The heart rate,

respiratory rate, and rectal temperature were within normal ranges. Feces were loose and the horse was mildly dehydrated. By rectal examination, a firm impaction could be palpated in the cecum. No sand was detected in the feces.

Laboratory findings

Eosinophils: $0.76 \times 10^3/mm^3$ (absolute eosinophilia)

McMaster: 40 strongyle EPG and 280 *Anoplocephala* eggs/gram. a modified egg counting technique for detecting tapeworm eggs using 30 grams of feces revealed a total of 563 *Anoplocephala* eggs

Abdominal tap: 35 g protein/L; leukocytes – 20×10^9 cells/l (elevated); differential count – 27.5% eosinophils, 21% neutrophils, 44% macrophages, and 7.5% lymphocytes

Questions

1 What diagnoses would you include in your differential list?

2 Which treatments would you recommend?

Handbook of Equine Parasite Control, Second Edition. Martin K. Nielsen and Craig R. Reinemeyer.
© 2018 John Wiley & Sons, Inc. Published 2018 by John Wiley & Sons, Inc.

Outcome

The horse continued to colic despite various treatments. The owner could not afford further treatment and the horse was euthanatized on February 4.

Necropsy

More than 300 tapeworms were found loose in the cecal contents. At the ileocecal junction, the mucosa was irregular and had lymphoid elevations protruding into the lumen. All recovered parasites were identified as *Anoplocephala perfoliata* based on morphologic criteria. In addition, three specimens of *Setaria equina* were recovered from the abdominal cavity. (The latter were the likely cause of the observed eosinophil counts both in the blood and the abdominal cavity.)

3 The owner wants to know if the horse was already infected with the parasites at the time of the previous colic episode in September. What is your opinion?

Herd management

Due to the nature of the case, the farm owner wished to investigate the level of tapeworm infection in the remainder of

Table C14.1 Serum ELISA results for horses in the herd.

Horse	O.D.
A	1.709
B	2.000
C	2.000
D	1.990
E	0.235
F	0.482
G	0.117
H	1.627

the herd. Eight adult riding horses were resident on the farm, and both serum and fecal samples were collected for tapeworm analysis. The tapeworm serum optic density (OD) values are presented in Table C14.1.

On the modified tapeworm egg count, only horse "A" had a positive tapeworm fecal result.

4 What is your interpretation of these results? Are the surviving horses at risk of developing similar clinical conditions?

5 What treatment recommendations would you offer to the herd manager?

Answers

1 **Clinical diagnoses:**
   Tapeworm infection with associated cecal impaction.
   Peritonitis.

   Differential diagnoses:
   Caecal invagination or other mechanical obstruction requiring surgery.
   Cyathostominosis.

2 Supportive therapy included intravenous fluids and analgesics; metamizole, butorphanol, and flunixin. Antibiotics: benzyl penicillin, gentamycin and metronidazole. The horse was eventually treated with praziquantel/ivermectin.

3 Tapeworms may interfere with local alimentary motility, could have contributed to the cecal impaction, and possibly have interfered with passage of ingesta through the ileum as well.

Adult tapeworms could have been established in this horse at the time of the first hospital admission in September. Most cestode infections are acquired during the grazing months, and burdens peak in autumn and early winter. The plain McMaster technique used for routine fecal egg counts lacks sensitivity for detecting tapeworm eggs (Chapter 9), so a cestode infection could have been missed on that occasion.

4 Considered *in toto*, the test results suggest that this herd is widely exposed to tapeworm infection. At the time of examination, however, only one horse had detectable egg-shedding. This suggests that several of the horses had recent exposure to tapeworms, but none had a worm burden approaching the magnitude of that in the fatal case. It was concluded in this particular case that other factors had rendered the horse more susceptible to tapeworms.

5 The remainder of the herd was treated with praziquantel before turn-out in spring. It was recommended that the entire herd be treated each autumn with a combination drug containing a macrocyclic lactone and praziquantel. For strongyle control, it was recommended that fecal samples be collected in the spring for FECRT and that selective therapy be implemented thereafter.

Case 15

Ivermectin Efficacy

History

A client asks you to evaluate the efficacy of ivermectin in a herd of Warmblood show jumpers. You perform pre- and post-treatment egg counts on nine adult horses in total. These horses were treated with ivermectin paste and post-treatment samples were collected 14 days later. A McMaster method with a detection limit of 20 EPG was used for both examinations; the respective strongylid egg counts are presented in Table C15.1.

Table C15.1 Pre- and post-treatment strongyle egg counts from a herd of horses treated with ivermectin.

Horse	Pre-treatment	Post-treatment
A	800	20
B	360	0
C	280	0
D	200	0
E	340	0
F	220	0
G	200	0
H	200	0
J	1320	1280

Questions

1 Calculate the fecal egg count reduction percentage for the herd.

2 What is your interpretation of the FECRT result?

3 What will you recommend to your client regarding future use of ivermectin in this herd?

Handbook of Equine Parasite Control, Second Edition. Martin K. Nielsen and Craig R. Reinemeyer.
© 2018 John Wiley & Sons, Inc. Published 2018 by John Wiley & Sons, Inc.

Answers

1 With horse J included, the calculated group FECR is 66.8%. If "J" were excluded from the data set, however, the FECR would be 99.2%.

2 Horse J is a clear outlier and should not be included in the FECR calculations. In all likelihood, "J" was either inadvertently skipped during treatment or perhaps it managed to reject its dose of paste unnoticed. Supporting this conclusion is the observation that none of the other horses exhibited signs of reduced efficacy. However, these results should be interpreted with caution, because all of the horses with 100% FECRs had low to moderate pre-treatment egg counts. A slight decrease in FECR therefore might not be detected because the detection limit of the McMaster was moderate (20 EPG). However, a few post-treatment egg counts of <20 EPG would not cause the group FECR to drop dramatically. It is also worth noting that the two horses with positive, post-treatment egg counts also had the highest pre-treatment egg counts. See Chapter 10 for a further discussion of interpreting FECRT.

Viewed comprehensively, this FECRT exercise detected no evidence of ivermectin resistance, but a more reliable estimate of IVM efficacy could be achieved by (a) including more horses with higher egg counts or (b) using an egg count technique with a lower detection limit, such as the FLOTAC, Mini-FLOTAC, FECPAK, Stoll, or Wisconsin (see Chapter 10).

3 The client should be advised to re-treat horse J (meticulously) with ivermectin and submit another post-treatment sample for evaluation of efficacy. In general, avermectins and milbemycins appear to maintain good efficacy in this herd, although future re-evaluations are warranted on an annual basis.

Case 16

Anthelmintic Treatments in Foals

History

A Thoroughbred farm deworms all foals by 2 months of age with a single dose of fenbendazole and then conducts egg counts at about 4 months of age. The 4-month egg counts are presented in Table C16.1. The manager has several questions for you.

Table C16.1 Fecal egg count results (eggs per gram) from a group of 4 month old foals.

Foal	Strongyle	Ascarid	Other	Foal	Strongyle	Ascarid	Other
1	12	16	0	20	0	0	0
2	17	1	0	21	0	0	0
3	0	0	0	22	3	0	0
4	0	0	0	23	0	0	0
5	0	0	0	24	0	0	1 *A. perfoliata*
6	32	7	0	25	0	0	0
7	2	0	0	26	0	0	0
8	0	0	0	27	3	29	0
9	0	3	0	28	0	0	0
10	0	11	0	29	8	12	0
11	0	10	0	30	0	0	0
12	96	0	0	31	9	0	0
13	0	0	0	32	0	0	0
14	0	0	31 *S. westeri*	33	0	0	0
15	0	0	0	34	4	0	0
16	22	8	0	35	0	0	0
17	0	0	0	36	11	0	0
18	0	0	0	37	8	91	0
19	19	4	0				

Handbook of Equine Parasite Control, Second Edition. Martin K. Nielsen and Craig R. Reinemeyer.
© 2018 John Wiley & Sons, Inc. Published 2018 by John Wiley & Sons, Inc.

Questions

1 He is concerned about tapeworms showing up this early (foal 24) and wants your advice.

2 He also tells you that they seem to be finding sporadic occurrences of *S. westeri* eggs in this age group and is asking for your treatment recommendations for this parasite.

3 Finally, he intends to treat all these foals prior to weaning at 5 months of age and wants you to recommend the most appropriate anthelmintic.

Answers

1 The prepatent period of tapeworms is longer than 4 months (Chapter 1) and patent infections with *A. perfoliata* should not develop in foals/weanlings until about 6 to 7 months of age. The most likely explanation of this observation is coprophagy, which is normal behavior in this age group.

2 Yes, sporadic infections with *S. westeri* do occur in this age group. These infections are unlikely to be lactogenically transmitted, but rather reflect orally or transcutaneously acquired larvae. These individuals that exhibit sporadic egg shedding can usually clear a *Strongyloides* infection without anthelmintic intervention, but both ivermectin (0.2 mg/kg) and oxibendazole (15 mg/kg) have label claims for efficacy against this parasite (Chapter 7).

3 Priority should be given to controlling ascarid parasites at this age, so the recommendation should be to treat with a benzimidazole again. Follow-up egg counts can be evaluated 2 weeks post-treatment to assess whether a strongyle-directed treatment should be considered prior to weaning. Ivermectin would be the most appropriate choice for this purpose.

Case 17

Ivermectin Egg Reappearance

History

You have been using ivermectin almost exclusively for a decade or more in a small string of Quarter Horse brood mares that you own in partnership with a good friend. You are both curious about the status of ivermectin in this herd because you heard recently in an on-line webinar that a shorter egg reappearance period (ERP) after ivermectin treatment could be interpreted as evidence of developing resistance to the drug. You both decide to evaluate the efficacy of ivermectin in this herd and to measure the ERP in a systematic fashion.

Nine mares with positive egg counts are selected and dewormed with ivermectin paste. At 7-day intervals during weeks 2 through 8 post-treatment, fecal samples are collected for quantitative analysis. The FEC results are presented in Table C17.1.

Table C17.1 Strongyle egg counts of fecal samples collected prior to and weekly after ivermectin treatment (McMaster technique with a detection limit of 25 EPG).

Pre-treatment	Week 2	Week 3	Week 4	Week 5	Week 6	Week 7	Week 8
225	0	0	0	0	25	25	25
875	0	0	25	50	25	100	175
700	0	0	0	0	50	150	250
200	0	0	0	0	0	0	25
650	0	0	0	25	75	50	100
975	0	0	0	25	50	200	150
400	0	0	0	0	0	25	0
350	0	0	0	0	25	50	100
1025	0	25	0	75	125	250	250

Questions

1 Calculate the weekly fecal egg count reductions (FECR) for this herd.

2 What is your interpretation regarding the current status of ivermectin efficacy in this group of mares?

3 What is your recommendation for future use of ivermectin?

Handbook of Equine Parasite Control, Second Edition. Martin K. Nielsen and Craig R. Reinemeyer.
© 2018 John Wiley & Sons, Inc. Published 2018 by John Wiley & Sons, Inc.

Answers

1 The FECR results are presented in Table C17.2.

2 The mean FECR for the group does not fall below an 85% cutoff (see Chapter 10) until week 7. However, the result for week 7 could be considered border line. Overall, this herd exhibits an ERP of 6 to 7 weeks for ivermectin, which is considered satisfactory. This collection of data indicates no signs of ivermectin resistance.

3 The client can keep using ivermectin for strongyle treatment. If he is motivated to monitor the efficacy of ivermectin in coming seasons, you could suggest performing the post-treatment egg counts one time in weeks 5 or 6.

Table C17.2 Calculated, weekly fecal egg count reductions (FECR) for individual horses after ivermectin treatment. Group total fecal egg counts and group FECRs are presented for each week post-treatment.

Pre-treatment	Week 2	Week 3	Week 4	Week 5	Week 6	Week 7	Week 8
5400	0	25	25	175	375	850	1,075
	100%	99.5%	99.5%	96.8%	93.1%	84.3%	80.1%

Case 18

Name That Worm

History

While evacuating the rectum of a 7 year old Standardbred mare in preparation for reproductive ultrasound, the vet noticed one fairly large (~3.5 cm), cream-colored nematode that was removed with the feces (Figure C18.1). After concluding the procedure, two similar worms were found adhering to his O.B. sleeve.

The mare had not been dewormed for 6 months and had exhibited no abnormal clinical signs. The owner requested a diagnosis and wanted to know about therapeutic and management recommendations.

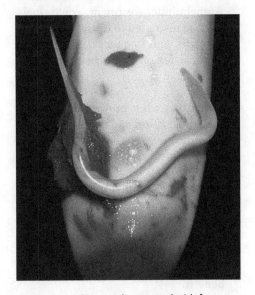

Figure C18.1 Nematode removed with feces.

Handbook of Equine Parasite Control, Second Edition. Martin K. Nielsen and Craig R. Reinemeyer.
© 2018 John Wiley & Sons, Inc. Published 2018 by John Wiley & Sons, Inc.

Questions

1 What is the parasitologic diagnosis?

2 Should other horses in the herd be screened?

3 Which anthelmintic(s) would you recommend?

4 The owner has heard that administering anthelmintics via rectal lavage should be effective against pinworms. Would you recommend this treatment, and if so which anthelmintics would you use and in which formulation?

Answers

1 Pinworm infection (*Oxyuris equi*). The observed specimens were likely adult females; males are much smaller and generally less numerous. These worms normally inhabit the dorsal colon as adults. Females are commonly seen on freshly passed feces. Historically, most pinworm infections have been observed in juvenile horses, but this parasite occurs more commonly in adult horses now.

2 Diagnostic screening would not provide many definitive answers. If one horse is infected, the remainder of the herd has probably been exposed. Pinworm infections are more likely in immature horses than in mature stock, but this historical pattern seems to be changing on many farms. Pinworms do not lay eggs in feces, so screening by flotation or quantitative procedures would be fairly useless. Pinworm eggs are best detected by the Scotch tape technique or by perianal scraping (see Chapter 9).

3 Recent reports suggest pinworm resistance to ivermectin (see Chapter 8), and pyrantel formulations have always had variable efficacy against this parasite. By default, benzimidazoles may be the best treatment option.

Stall hygiene would have limited benefit for preventing infections. Anthelmintic treatment could logically be restricted to horses with clinical signs, and frequent bathing of the perianal region might help to relieve pruritus.

4 Given that adult pinworms reside in the dorsal colon and females are only encountered in the rectum while migrating to the anal area to deliver their egg package (Chapter 1), a rectal lavage is unlikely to offer any reduction of pinworm burdens. It should be noted that any females encountered in the rectum will likely die immediately after laying their eggs, so lavage treatment offers little benefit.

Case 19

Parasite Control for Yearlings

History

A local trainer contacts you in late winter with questions about deworming her charges prior to the approaching grazing season. All of her horses are youngsters, ranging from weanlings to a 3 year old. The results of recent quantitative fecal exams are presented in Table C19.1.

Table C19.1 Ascarid and strongylid fecal egg counts (EPG) of young horses in training.

Horse	Age*	Strongyle	Ascarid
A	1.5	350	0
B	1.5	500	0
C	1.5	500	0
D	0.5	300	0
E	0.5	150	150
F	0.5	0	100
G	1	200	50
H	3	0	0

*Expressed in years.

Questions

1 Based on the egg counts, would you treat any of these horses?
   A If so, which ones?

2 List the anthelmintics that you would consider using.
   A Provide the rationale for your recommendations.

Handbook of Equine Parasite Control, Second Edition. Martin K. Nielsen and Craig R. Reinemeyer.
© 2018 John Wiley & Sons, Inc. Published 2018 by John Wiley & Sons, Inc.

Answers

1 None of the egg counts are alarmingly high. In fact, the strongyle egg counts are relatively low, considering the age of the hosts. However, it should be remembered that egg counts are often lower during winter months. The presence of ascarid eggs in horses of this age group is not unexpected. Anthelmintic treatments could be considered, but it primarily depends on when these horses were last treated.

   A A major consideration regarding treatment at this time is the presence of ascarids in three foals (E, F, G), especially the possibility of small intestinal impaction. If these horses had been treated for strongyles in the fall, and they currently appear healthy, strongyle treatments could wait until spring, when active translation can occur on pasture.

2 For ascarid treatment, a benzimidazole is recommended. If the trainer elects to treat for strongyles, ivermectin and/or moxidectin would be a rational choice, but pyrantel could also be used if known to be efficacious.

   A The risk of small intestinal impaction appears to be considerably less with benzimidazole treatments compared to drugs with paralytic modes of action (see Chapter 7). In healthy horses, the primary reason for a strongyle treatment is to decrease egg shedding. Benzimidazole resistance is extremely prevalent in cyathostomins and cannot be expected to work, unless a fecal egg count reduction test has indicated otherwise. Pyrantel could work on some farms, but again, the local efficacy needs to be verified. Moxidectin is particularly useful for larvicidal therapy, treatment of clinical cases of parasitic disease, and treatment of extreme high contaminators. Ivermectin/moxidectin resistance may be an emerging problem among cyathostomins, so it is recommended to monitor their efficacy on a routine basis.

Case 20

Reaction to Treatment

History

During May in Louisiana, USA, a client deworms her 10 year old Paint gelding with generic ivermectin in preparation for pending competitions. Two days later, she notices some significant swelling along the ventral midline and the horse is rubbing its chest on the stall door and its withers against trees in the pasture. None of her other horses are exhibiting similar behavior.

Clinical presentation

Upon closer examination, the dependent edema involves areas of discrete hair

loss with slight crusting along the ventral midline. Multiple, small lesions are also noted on the face, neck, and withers, but these are limited to slight hair loss and focal accumulations of gray scales. A cursory exam reveals that several pasture mates have similar lesions, although none are exhibiting severe pruritus.

The show season for this horse has abruptly ended and the owner wants to know if the manufacturer has any legal liability for this obvious allergic reaction to ivermectin.

Questions

1 Can you give a plausible parasitological explanation for the observed reactions?

2 How could you achieve a definitive diagnosis?

3 What are your treatment and future management recommendations?

Answers

1 The lesions in all the pastured horses are consistent with *Onchocerca* spp. infection. The focal host reactions develop in response to microfilarial stages in the dermis. Microfilariae are killed by macrocyclic lactones, and pruritus, edema, and local inflammation of the dermis are common reactions to dying worms, not a reaction to the anthelmintic itself (Chapter 7).

Handbook of Equine Parasite Control, Second Edition. Martin K. Nielsen and Craig R. Reinemeyer.
© 2018 John Wiley & Sons, Inc. Published 2018 by John Wiley & Sons, Inc.

All horses on the premises should be similarly exposed to *Onchocerca* infection, which is transmitted by the bite of arthropod vectors (*Culicoides* spp.).

2 Diagnosis can be confirmed by demonstrating motile microfilariae in skin biopsies (see Chapter 9). Because microfilariae in the treated horse are probably dead, diagnostic efforts would be more productive if skin biopsies from one of the untreated pasture mates were examined.

3 Macrocyclic lactone treatment is usually sufficient to kill the microfilarial stages and alleviate the skin lesions. The adult worms, which reside in deep connective tissues, are not killed by ivermectin, but apparently are rendered infertile for intervals of several months. Microfilarial production eventually resumes, so intermittent macrocyclic lactone treatment may be required to prevent recurring skin lesions. Measures intended to limit *Culicoides* exposure (*e.g.*, nocturnal stabling, window screens, overhead fans) are useful adjuncts for preventing infection.

Case 21

Anthelmintic Toxicosis?

History

A large Quarter Horse breeding farm experienced a sudden onset of neurological symptoms in three foals aged 2 to 3 months of age. The foals presented with ataxia, dyspnea, depression, tremors, and weakness. Two of them had to be euthanized for ethical reasons, while the third foal was only mildly affected and recovered after hospitalization and supportive therapy. The farm manager informed the veterinarian that they had just dewormed the mares with moxidectin oral gel. The foals were not dewormed at this time, but one of the staff members had noticed that the foals had been drinking water out of the same bucket as the dams and speculated that the moxidectin gel had been transferred to the foals through the water. The local veterinary diagnostic laboratory measured the concentration of moxidectin in the brain tissue in both foals and found it to be about ten times elevated compared to correctly dosed horses 24 hours post-treatment.

Questions

1 Are the described symptoms consistent with moxidection toxicosis?

2 Is the explanation offered by the farm staff plausible? Why/why not?

Answers

1 Yes, these symptoms have been described in foals with moxidectin toxicosis (Chapter 7). Furthermore, the elevated concentration of moxidectin in the brain tissue strongly supports this diagnosis.

2 No. The elevated brain concentrations of moxidectin suggest a severe overdose of this anthelmintic and would not support the theory of contaminated water. For this to happen, the mare would have had to spit the entire dose into the water bucket and the foal would have had to ingest the entire dose. This is highly unlikely to happen in one foal and should be considered virtually impossible in three foals. The veterinarian told the farm manager that another explanation should be sought.

Handbook of Equine Parasite Control, Second Edition. Martin K. Nielsen and Craig R. Reinemeyer.
© 2018 John Wiley & Sons, Inc. Published 2018 by John Wiley & Sons, Inc.

After some interrogation of farm personnel, it turned out that the mares had been treated by squirting the entire dose of moxidectin gel on to their grain instead of administering it orally. Since the foals were present with the mares at the time and had started developing a taste for the concentrate diet, their mothers let them eat from the buckets first, which led to this unfortunate event.

Case 22

Deworming Program Adjustment?

History

A Standardbred farm produces about 30 foals every year. Foals are dewormed with fenbendazole (10 mg/kg) at 1.5 months of age and then followed up with ivermectin (0.2 mg/kg) 5 weeks later. The mares are dewormed every 8 weeks in a rotational fashion. The farm has had no history of poor growth or ill-thrift in their foals. A 4 month old foal was euthanized for a traumatic orthopedic lesion and hundreds of mature ascarids were found in the small intestine at necropsy. This foal was in good body condition and was growing well, with no indications of parasite infection prior to euthanasia.

Question

1   The veterinarian wants to know if the treatment program should be adjusted and, if so, how.

Answer

1   The worms encountered in a 4-month-old foal are not a big surprise as this is the age of peak ascarid burdens. It is also important to emphasize to the owner that all the foals are clinically healthy and the foal in question was euthanatized for unrelated reasons. Therefore, the information presented here does not provide a reason for being overly concerned about ascarids *per se*. However, there are a few adjustments to consider:

A   The fenbendazole treatment administered at 6 weeks of age may be a little early, considering that a considerable proportion of ascarids would be in the migrating phase at this point in time and the intestinal stages would be very young (Chapter 1). The recommendation is to treat foals at 2–3 months of age (Chapter 12).

B   The ivermectin treatment administered at 11 weeks of age was unlikely to be very effective, given the world-wide findings of resistance to this drug in *Parascaris* spp. (Chapter 8). Foals around 3 months of age are primarily parasitized by ascarids, and with little or no reduction of worm burdens following an ineffective treatment,

Handbook of Equine Parasite Control, Second Edition. Martin K. Nielsen and Craig R. Reinemeyer.
© 2018 John Wiley & Sons, Inc. Published 2018 by John Wiley & Sons, Inc.

this foal could have accumulated a large worm burden just a few weeks later. Another treatment with a benzimidazole would have been a more appropriate choice.

C There is no justification for keeping the mares on an 8 week rotational deworming schedule (Chapter 12). Two treatments a year should suffice for the large majority of brood mares, depending on climatic conditions and the proportion of high strongyle shedders present in the herd. Furthermore, there is no benefit to rotational deworming (Chapter 7).

Glossary

Abdominocentesis A procedure to collect fluid from the abdominal cavity ("belly tap")

Accuracy A measure of proximity between a diagnostic result and the "true" value

Adulticidal Treatment that kills adult worms

Agonist Compound that has the same effect as a given substance

Anaphylaxis A systemic allergic reaction

Anemia Low concentration of red blood cells

Anoplocephalinae The subfamily of tapeworms infecting horses

Antagonist Compound that has the opposite effect as a given substance

Anthelmintic Dewormer; compound with efficacy against helminth parasites

Arteritis Inflammation of arteries

Arthropod Invertebrates with an exoskeleton and jointed legs (examples include insects, spiders, ticks and mites)

Ascarid Large nematode parasite; "roundworms"

Ascaridoidea The superfamily of ascarids infecting various domestic animals and humans

Baermann A sedimentation procedure used to diagnose parasites

Buccal capsule Oral cavity/mouthparts of nematodes used for identification

Cephalic Associated with the head region

Cestode Tapeworm

Conjunctivitis Inflammation of the mucosal membranes around the eyes

Coproantigen Antigens presented in fecal matter

Coproculture Method used to grow and recover larval stages from fecal samples

Coprophagy Habit of eating feces; normal behavior in foals

Copulatory bursa Male reproductive structure in some nematodes

Cryptic species Species that look alike but are genetically different

Cutaneous Regarding the skin

Cuticle A non-cellular, membranous protective covering of worms and larvae

Cyathostominae Small strongyle subfamily

Cyathostomins Parasites belonging to the Cyathostominae

Cysticercoid The infective, larval stage of anoplocephalid tapeworms

Definitive host The natural, final host for a parasite, in which sexual reproduction takes place

Dermatitis Inflammation of the skin

Dipterans An order of insects with two pairs of wings; flies

Edema An accumulation of fluid within a tissue

Egg reappearance period The time elapsed from anthelmintic treatment to positive strongyle egg counts

Embryonated egg Egg with a developed larva inside

Handbook of Equine Parasite Control, Second Edition. Martin K. Nielsen and Craig R. Reinemeyer.
© 2018 John Wiley & Sons, Inc. Published 2018 by John Wiley & Sons, Inc.

Encystment Encapsulation of cyathostomin larvae within the mucosa

Eosinophilia Elevated numbers of eosinophil granulocytes in the blood

Eukaryotic Animals with a cell nucleus, as opposed to prokaryotic

Excystment Process of cyathostomin larvae leaving mucosal cysts

Exsheathe Process of third-stage larva losing its outer cuticle

Extra-label Use of a medicine in a dosage, animal species, or target indication for which it is not approved

Fecundity Egg-producing capacity of female worms

Fibrinolysis The breakdown of fibrin in blood clots

Filarioid Parasite belonging to the Filarioidea

Filarioidea Superfamily of threadlike nematodes that produce microfilariae and are often transmitted by arthropods

Genus, genera Taxonomic division between family and species

Gingival Related to the tissues around the teeth; "gums"

Hematogenous Derived from or carried in the blood stream

Hematophagous Organism that ingests blood

Hemorrhage Bleeding

Hypoproteinemia Lowered concentration of protein in the blood

Infarction Tissue death due to inadequate blood supply

Instar Larval stage of a bot fly (*Gasterophilus* spp.) or any dipteran

Intermediate host Host in which a parasite develops before infecting a final host

Intussusception One segment of intestine telescoping into the next

Ischemia Restriction of blood supply causing a shortage of oxygen in a given tissue

Keratitis Inflammation of the cornea (eye)

Lactogenic Related to the milk

Laparotomy Surgical procedure in which the abdominal cavity is opened

Larvicidal Treatment that kills larval parasites

Lieberkühn, glands of Digestive glands found throughout the intestine

Lingual Related to the tongue

Luminal Related to the hollow space inside the intestine

Microfilariae First larval stage of filarioid parasites

Molt The transition between parasitic stages

Monospecific Infection with just one species of parasite present

Mucocutaneous Junction between mucosal and cutaneous (skin) surfaces

Mucosa Mucous membrane, usually delicate and moist (*e.g.*, inside the mouth, alimentary tract, vagina

Necrotic Pertaining to tissue death

Nematode Roundworm

Neutrophilia Elevated numbers of neutrophil granulocytes in the blood

Oestrid Parasite belonging to the botfly family (Oestridae)

Oncosphere The embryo stage of a tapeworm; precursor of a scolex

Oribatid Mite belonging to the Oribatidae

Oribatidae Family of mites that can act as intermediate hosts for equine tapeworms

Ostertagiosis Disease caused by *Ostertagia* nematodes in cattle

Oxyuroid Parasite belonging to the Oxyuroidea.

Oxyuroidea Superfamily of pinworm parasites

Pancreatitis Inflammation of the pancreas

Paratenic host Host in which a parasite is carried without any further development ("biological taxi")

Parenchyma The functional tissue of an organ

Parenteral Administered or occurring outside the gastrointestinal tract

Patency Egg production during a parasitic infection

Pathogenic Causing tissue damage/ pathological lesions

Pathognomonic Signs or findings unique to a specific disease

Periodontitis Inflammation of the deep tissues around the teeth

Peristalsis Spasmodic contractions of the alimentary tract

Peritonitis Inflammation of the tissues lining the abdominal cavity

Precision Measure of similarity or proximity of repeated measures

Prepatent period Time elapsed from infection to the egg-shedding (*i.e.*, "patent") stage

Proglottids Tapeworm segments

Protozoa Large group of single-celled, eukaryotic parasites

Pseudomembrane A contiguous layer of exudate resembling a membrane

Purulent Condition containing or discharging pus

Refugia That portion of a parasite population that is not exposed to treatment

Resilience Host capability to harbor parasites without being affected

Retroperitoneal Outside or beneath the peritoneal membrane

Rhabditoid Parasite belonging to the Rhabditoidea

Rhabditoidea Superfamily of nematodes, many of which are free-living

Scolex The "head" or anterior end of a tapeworm

Spasmodic Causing or involving spasms; often used in reference to intestinal spasms as a mechanism for colic

Spiruroid Parasite belonging to the Spiruroidea

Spiruroidea Superfamily of arthropod-borne parasites

Strobila The segmented part (body) of a tapeworm

Strongyle Member of the nematode family Strongylidae; synonym to strongylid and strongyloid.

Strongylid Synonym to strongyle and strongyloid

Strongylidae Nematode family containing large (Strongylinae) and small (Cyathostominae) strongyles

Strongylinae Subfamily of large strongyles

Strongyloid Synonym to strongylid and strongyle

Submucosa Layer of tissue beneath a mucosal membrane

Tegument The outer layer ("skin") of tapeworms and flukes

Thrombi Blood clots

Thromboembolism Blood clots which move about in the blood stream

Toxicosis Intoxication or poisoning

Transabdominal Through or across the abdominal wall

Transcutaneous Through or across the skin

Transmural Through or across a wall or septum

Trematode Taxonomic division containing all fluke parasites

Trichonemes Outdated term for cyathostomins.

Trichostrongyloid Parasite belonging to the Trichostrongyloidea.

Trichostrongyloidea Superfamily of strongylid parasites infecting ruminants

Vector An organism that transmits a parasite or other organism to an animal

Volvulus Torsion or twisting of stomach or intestine

Index

Handbook of Equine Parasite Control, Second Edition. Martin K. Nielsen and Craig R. Reinemeyer.
© 2018 John Wiley & Sons, Inc. Published 2018 by John Wiley & Sons, Inc.